OECD Health Policy Studies

Care Needed

IMPROVING THE LIVES OF PEOPLE WITH DEMENTIA

OECD
BETTER POLICIES FOR BETTER LIVES

This work is published under the responsibility of the Secretary-General of the OECD. The opinions expressed and arguments employed herein do not necessarily reflect the official views of OECD member countries.

This document, as well as any data and any map included herein, are without prejudice to the status of or sovereignty over any territory, to the delimitation of international frontiers and boundaries and to the name of any territory, city or area.

Please cite this publication as:
OECD (2018), *Care Needed: Improving the Lives of People with Dementia*, OECD Health Policy Studies, OECD Publishing, Paris.
http://dx.doi.org/10.1787/9789264085107-en

ISBN 978-92-64-08509-1 (print)
ISBN 978-92-64-08510-7 (PDF)

Series: OECD Health Policy Studies
ISSN 2074-3181 (print)
ISSN 2074-319X (online)

The statistical data for Israel are supplied by and under the responsibility of the relevant Israeli authorities. The use of such data by the OECD is without prejudice to the status of the Golan Heights, East Jerusalem and Israeli settlements in the West Bank under the terms of international law.

Photo credits: Cover © Yurchanka Siarhei/Shutterstock and Macrovector/Freepik for the pictos Graphic design by Vif Argent

Corrigenda to OECD publications may be found on line at: *www.oecd.org/about/publishing/corrigenda.htm*.

Foreword

As populations continue to age, the number of people living with dementia in OECD countries is expected to rise from an estimated 19 million today to 40.9 million by 2050. Until a cure for dementia is found, this will have large human and financial implications.

Improving the lives of people living with dementia is both a moral necessity and an economic imperative. Too many people with dementia are not diagnosed, and for those who are, a dementia diagnosis can be devastating. Stigma towards dementia remains too common, and many people are left to manage their condition without adequate access to health and social care services that could help them. The cost for individuals and their families is huge – 40-75% of the total dementia care cost. There are high costs for health and care systems from poor quality care, too. Think for example of the large number of hospitalisations of dementia patients that could be avoided through better investment in prevention and care co-ordination. There is growing evidence that prevention to address risk factors for several chronic conditions is also good for preventing dementia. Yet health systems across the OECD only devote less than 3% of health spending to prevention.

In recent years, policy attention towards dementia has grown. At the national level, many OECD countries have focussed efforts on improving the quality of care that people with dementia receive and raising awareness in communities through dementia friends initiatives. Several countries have developed dementia care plans. At the global level, initiatives such as the G8 Summit on Dementia in London (United Kingdom) in 2013 and the creation of the World Dementia Council, among others, are encouraging signs that the global community has taken notice of this pressing issue and is committed to developing innovative solutions to tackle dementia. The OECD has been an active voice in many of these global efforts. The 2015 report *Addressing Dementia: The OECD Response* already developed a framework for the key objectives of dementia policy.

Yet despite these efforts, we are still failing too many people with dementia. Significant gaps remain in access to and quality of services. Close to 70% of nursing home residents have some form of cognitive impairment, yet staff has often not received training to adequately treat the symptoms of advanced dementia and significant inappropriate use of drugs for behavioural and psychotic symptoms of dementia remains. Data and measurement for dementia are weak and frustrate efforts to monitor progress. Fewer than 40% of countries, for example, are able to estimate their national diagnosis rate.

This report presents an exhaustive look into what OECD countries have done to improve care for dementia across the pathway of the condition. New data collected underscore how far many countries still have to go to ensure that people living with dementia receive high-quality care. In evaluating country progress, this report draws attention to how dementia care continues to be held back by major knowledge and measurement gaps. The findings of this report will help countries further improve how they care for people with dementia today, and set the groundwork for high-quality care in the years to come.

Acknowledgements

This report was prepared by the OECD Health Division. It was coordinated by Tim Atkins (previously with the OECD and currently at the Care Quality Commission, United Kingdom) and Elina Suzuki, and benefited from the expertise and participation of experts within the Health Division as well as country delegates and experts. The report was written by Tim Atkins and Elina Suzuki. Chapter 3 was also co-authored by Ivy Wong, Julie Dunning, Dr. Geoffrey Anderson, Dr. Onil Bhattacharyya, Dr. Samir Sinha, Dara Gordon, Dilzayn Panjwani and Sara Shearkhani, who are all part of BeACCoN (Ontario's Network in Primary and Integrated Health Care Innovations), as well as Ishtar Al-Shammari of the International Consortium for Health Outcomes Measurement (ICHOM) in London, United Kingdom.

The findings of this report were strongly informed by work to pilot dementia quality of care indicators undertaken by the OECD Health Care Quality Indicators (HCQI) Expert Group. The authors would like to thank the country delegates and experts who provided responses to the scoping survey and questionnaire, as well as those who participated in interviews for the report. The report also benefited from the very helpful comments received by delegates from the OECD Health Committee meeting.

The completion of this report was made possible through the generous support of the United Kingdom. We especially thank David Nuttall and Simon Dowlman of the Department of Health, United Kingdom, for their feedback during the drafting of the report. The authors are also deeply grateful to Paola Barbarino, Chris Lynch, Glen Rees and James Smith of Alzheimer's Disease International for their very valuable feedback on multiple iterations of the report.

The authors are also grateful to the contributions of the staff from the OECD Health Division. In particular, the authors would like to recognise Ana Llena-Nozal, who leads the work on long-term care, and Emily Hewlett, for their very helpful comments on multiple drafts of the report. Thanks also go to Lucy Hulett, Eileen Rocard and Duniya Dedeyn for their administrative support and help in preparing the manuscript for publication. We are very grateful to Francesca Colombo, Head of the Health Division, for supervising the preparation of this report and providing useful comments on various drafts. Thank you as well to Monika Queisser, Head of the Social Policy Division, for her insightful comments. We also thank Stefano Scarpetta and Mark Pearson, Director and Deputy Director of Employment, Labour and Social Affairs at the OECD for their guidance and extensive comments on various versions of the report.

Table of contents

Tables

Figures

Boxes

Acronyms and abbreviations

ACP	Advance care planning
AD	Advance directive
ADL	Activities of daily living
BPSD	Behavioural and psychological symptoms of dementia
CM	Case management
CST	Cognitive stimulation therapy
DB	Disability benefits
DBMAS	Dementia Behaviour Management Advisory Service
DKK	Danish Kroner
EU	European Union
EUR	Euros
FINGER	Finnish Geriatric Intervention Study to Prevent Cognitive Impairment and Disability
GBP	British Pound
HABC	Healthy Aging Brain Center
HELP	Hospital Elder Life Program
ICD	International Classification of Diseases
ICHOM	International Consortium for Health Outcomes Measurement
LTC	Long-term care
MAIA	Maisons pour l'Autonomie et l'Intégration des Malades Alzheimer
MMSE	Mini mental state exam
MoCA	Montreal Cognitive Exam
MOOC	Massive open online course
NHS	National Health Service
NICE	National Institute for Health and Care Excellence
NOK	Norwegian Kroner
NRR	Net replacement rate
OECD	Organisation for Economic Co-operation and Development
PPT	Pedagogical and Psychological Service
REACH	Resources for Enhancing Alzheimer's Caregiving Health
UPI	Unique patient identifier
USD	United States Dollar
WHO	World Health Organization

Executive summary

Dementia is a dreadful disease and a growing global challenge. The number of people living with dementia across the OECD reached nearly 19 million people in 2017, while millions of family members and friends provide care and support to loved ones with the condition throughout their lives. Beyond the personal and emotional toll of dementia, its financial costs are vast. The worldwide health and social costs of dementia were estimated to reach USD 1 trillion per year in 2018. Dementia is strongly associated with age. This makes the ageing of the population in many OECD countries the main factor associated with the growing dementia prevalence. As the share of the population aged above 80 years continues to rise, and until a cure or disease modifying treatment is found, the number of people living with dementia will continue to grow, and is likely to reach nearly 41 million people in the OECD by 2050.

Despite significant research efforts, much about the condition remains a mystery. No treatments have yet been developed that can effectively cure or halt the progression of dementia. Many recent late stage clinical trial failures have frustrated efforts and investment by the pharmaceutical industry. Further, today, too many people living with dementia go without a diagnosis. Even when they may be diagnosed, care systems are often fragmented, and the stigma surrounding dementia has led many people to believe that nothing can be done.

Yet the lack of a cure does not mean that there are no options. A range of beneficial services are available that can improve the health and quality of life of people living with dementia. However, in many cases, too few people have been able to access them. OECD countries urgently need to improve access to and quality of these services.

In recent years, dementia has received growing attention as governments begin to recognise the scope of the challenge ahead. As many as 22 OECD countries have developed national plans and strategies for addressing dementia, and have moved to make diagnosis and follow-up care more accessible and of higher quality. Treatment and care services can be further improved, and better monitoring and comparing of processes and outcomes will play an important role.

This report provides a detailed look at how OECD countries currently care for people living with dementia throughout their lives, from when they receive a diagnosis to the end of their lives. It lays out a number of key findings and lessons that help inform care for people with dementia:

Most countries remain poorly equipped to identify dementia

- Identifying dementia is important to developing and executing an effective response. A dementia diagnosis is one crucial step in accessing care and support, and receiving a timely diagnosis is important to take advantage of available treatment and care. Yet fewer than 40% of countries are able to estimate diagnosis rates nationally, and only two countries (Denmark and the United Kingdom) have set specific targets to improve diagnosis rates.

- Primary care serves as the first point of contact for people concerned about memory problems in 26 OECD countries. However, physicians average just 12 hours of dementia training during medical school, and very few countries provide financial or other incentives to encourage dementia-related training and continued professional development. This means that in many cases, primary care doctors are poorly prepared to diagnose dementia and correctly identify only around 50-75% of dementia cases.
- A firm diagnosis requires access to specialists, which is uneven across countries. The density of specialists who diagnose dementia varies more than three-fold across the OECD. At least 25 OECD countries have set up specialist centres called memory clinics to help with diagnosis. However, the characteristics and accessibility of these clinics are very heterogeneous. Only five countries (Denmark, France, the Netherlands, Switzerland, and the United Kingdom [England]) have developed or are in the process of developing guidelines and standards for the care delivered through these specialty centres.
- Data on dementia and dementia care remain extremely limited and can hamper efforts to improve quality of care and outcomes. Basic information, such as diagnosis rates, remains restricted even in countries with otherwise strong health data infrastructure. Just eight OECD countries measure diagnosis rates for dementia on a national level.
- Many OECD countries are seeking to improve the data landscape by linking data from different national datasets. However, important areas of the health system are frequently excluded from regular data linking. Many of the less frequently linked data sets include areas of the health system, such as primary care and long-term care, that are paramount for monitoring and improving dementia care. Some 45% of countries can link primary care with other data sources, but just 9% reported regularly doing so to monitor health care quality and performance. Five OECD countries (Canada, Finland, Israel, Korea, and the United Kingdom) regularly link long-term care data with hospital and mortality data, while only Korea and the United Kingdom regularly link primary care data with other data sources.

Initiatives to make communities inclusive and safe for people with dementia are fragmented

- Many people with dementia wish to live at home, and with the proper support they are often able to do so long after they have been diagnosed. Over 90% of OECD countries have developed at least some dementia-friendly community initiative to reduce stigma and improve the community response to people living with dementia. They include services such as social services, police forces and pharmacies, as well as training local and national businesses on how to engage with people living with dementia.
- Governments can play an important role in bringing attention to dementia-friendly activities. In most cases, however, such programmes remain ad-hoc and availability varies dramatically within countries, with just two countries (Japan and the

United Kingdom) having developed explicit targets related to dementia-friendly communities.

- Informal carers provide the majority of dementia care, with the costs of informal care estimated to represent between 40-75% of the total costs of caring for dementia. Caring for a person with dementia is more strenuous than many other types of caring. Carer support interventions have most often been designed for informal carers more broadly, and do not necessarily focus on the needs of dementia carers, whose needs can be greater than those caring for people with other conditions.
- The availability of respite care and training opportunities remains weak in many countries. In most cases, the availability of respite care depends on community capacity, and programmes are infrequently tailored to the needs of people with dementia and their carers. Offering more dementia-specific respite, such as respite holiday care programmes offered in Austria, can allow carers to relax while also being assured that their loved ones are being well cared for.
- Navigating the health and social care services available to people with dementia and their families can be difficult. Care co-ordination pathways to help people better access disparate services are particularly important for people with complex or rare cases of dementia. At least six OECD countries – Australia, Denmark, Estonia, France, the Netherlands, and Norway – have developed specialised care pathways for people with early or complex dementia.

The quality of care for people with advanced dementia is often poor and can result in worse health outcomes

- New data collected for this report confirm that the quality of care for people with advanced dementia remains in many cases poor. Despite widespread clinical agreement that antipsychotic medications should not be used to manage most difficult behaviour in dementia, rates of antipsychotic prescribing vary by a factor of more than two across the OECD. On average, one in twenty people aged 65 and over receives a prescription of antipsychotics across OECD countries.
- While dementia-specific training for formal care staff is available, incentives to encourage care workers to improve their dementia management skills remain the exception rather than the rule. Just four countries (Denmark, the Netherlands, Norway, and Sweden) have developed financial incentives targeted to care facilities or local authorities for further dementia training. Frameworks to recognise dementia care competencies, such as those developed in New Zealand and the United Kingdom (England), can help to better monitor the skills level of care workers and identify where further training is needed.
- The majority of people with dementia in care facilities continue to live in homes that are not designed for the needs of people with dementia, despite the fact that close to 70% of nursing home residents have some form of cognitive impairment. Only four countries – Denmark, Ireland, Norway, and the United Kingdom (England) – have developed design guidelines and advice to make care facilities more suitable for the needs of people with dementia.
- In recent years, a number of innovative residential care models have emerged. Innovative arrangements usually comprise of living environments where people

with dementia share a home with other residents, their families and staff, and can include small-scale living communities, multi-generational homes, and dementia villages. Yet spaces for people with dementia in innovative facilities are severely limited in every OECD country and facilities that provide the latest models of care are often private and very costly to patients.

- Inappropriate care can result in unnecessary or avoidable visits to the hospital, which can lead to even worse health outcomes for people with dementia. In some hospitals, people with dementia make up a quarter of all patients, but many are admitted for other illnesses or accidents without the hospital aware of their condition. Moreover, hospitals are not aware that a patient has dementia in most cases, even where a patient has already received a diagnosis. This can compromise their ability to deliver proper care for people with dementia. Improving hospital coding will help to better determine the care people with dementia receive, as well as to track and support efforts to reduce hospital (re)admissions.

Chapter 1. Key findings and conclusion

This chapter summarises the main findings of the report and explains the methodology used. It provides an overview of the state of dementia in OECD countries. In discussing the impact of dementia in OECD countries today and in the years to come, it makes the case for why greater attention to the condition and more concerted policy efforts are needed.

The statistical data for Israel are supplied by and under the responsibility of the relevant Israeli authorities. The use of such data by the OECD is without prejudice to the status of the Golan Heights, East Jerusalem and Israeli settlements in the West Bank under the terms of international law.

Nearly 19 million people across the OECD are living with dementia. Many more are affected by the disease: millions of family members and friends provide care or otherwise support their loved ones throughout their lives. Receiving a dementia diagnosis remains a shattering experience. Until a cure or disease-modifying treatment for dementia is developed, the progress of the disease cannot be slowed or stopped. Nevertheless, the quality of life and level of impairment that people experience can be improved. OECD countries already offer a range of treatments and services that can improve the lives of people with dementia, even in the absence of a cure. Medications, psychosocial interventions, dementia-friendly community initiatives and high-quality health and long-term care services can help people with dementia live more independently and maintain a higher level of wellbeing.

However, significant barriers to access remain and many people with dementia simply do not get the care they need to improve their lives or the lives of those close to them. Furthermore, many millions of cases of dementia go undiagnosed or are diagnosed late. Even when people receive services, these may fail to fully address their needs, and outcomes can be poor.

This report presents the state of the art in comparing dementia treatment and care, sets out estimates of the burden of dementia – diagnosed and undiagnosed – across OECD countries, reports on the state of dementia care across the OECD, and identifies the policies and practices that have been put in place to improve the quality of life for individuals living with dementia and their families. It builds on previous OECD work on dementia care, in particular *Addressing Dementia: the OECD Response*, which gave an overview of the evidence around dementia care and identified ten key objectives that all countries should consider when setting dementia policy (OECD, 2015a). This report deepens the analysis by comparing how these objectives are being addressed in different countries, both in terms of the policies that are being implemented and the outcomes that are being achieved. This report compares dementia care in OECD countries, and explores how better comparisons can be made in the future.

The report shows that countries have enhanced their efforts to provide high-quality dementia care during diagnosis, early and advanced dementia, but improving measurement is necessary for enhancements in care quality and outcomes for people with dementia. Chapter 2 presents an overview of recent efforts in countries to diagnose dementia and document and track people with dementia in the health system. It highlights in particular that diagnosis rates for dementia are low and efforts to expand diagnosis are often aimed at physicians underprepared to handle the job. Chapter 3 finds that while there is a growing body of good practice for community-based care, care co-ordination, dementia-friendly initiatives and support for informal carers must be further developed and more regularly measured to further progress. Finally, the research in Chapter 4 reveals that quality of care for advanced dementia remains poor, including high rates of antipsychotic prescribing which remain widespread despite the fact that such approaches are widely discouraged across the OECD.

1.1. Dementia will have a growing human and financial cost to society

1.1.1. Population ageing means dementia prevalence will continue to rise

Encompassing a range of health conditions, *dementia* refers to symptoms of memory and cognitive difficulties that can eventually interfere with the everyday life and activities of people living with dementia. While Alzheimer's disease is the most common form of dementia, other diseases exhibit similar symptoms, including vascular dementia, dementia with Lewy bodies, and Parkinson's disease.

Despite significant research efforts, much about dementia remains unknown. While it is clear that dementia does not represent a necessary outcome of ageing, dementia prevalence rises rapidly with age: while just over 2% of people between 65-69 years live with dementia, prevalence rises to over 40% for those aged over 90 (Figure 1.1).

Figure 1.1. Prevalence of dementia across all OECD countries, by age group

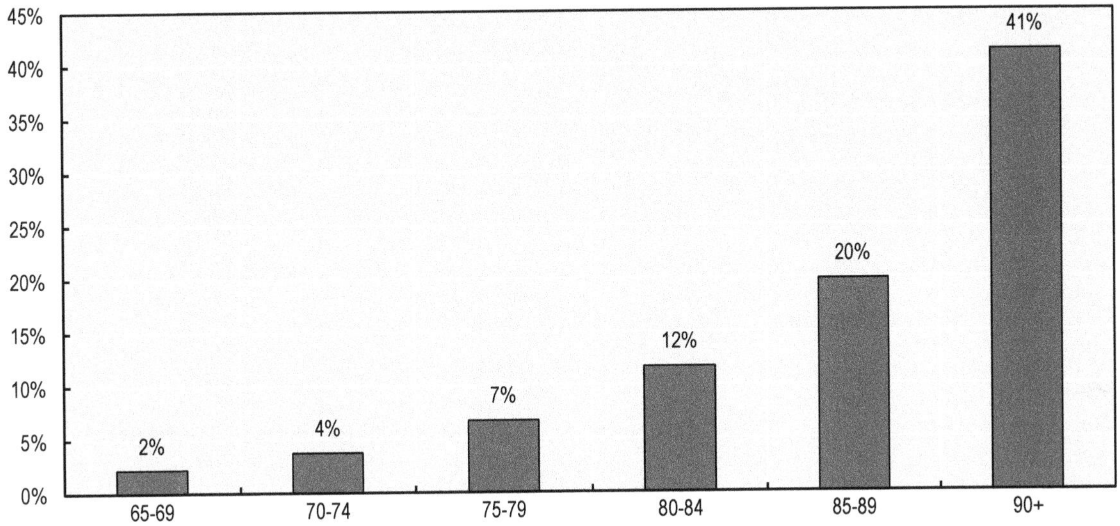

Source: *OECD Health Statistics 2017*, http://dx.doi.org/10.1787/health-data-en.

StatLink http://dx.doi.org/10.1787/888933735025

This makes the rapid ageing of the population in many OECD countries particularly relevant for dementia. The share of the population aged over 65 in OECD countries has risen quickly in recent years, and will continue to grow in the coming decades. On average, the proportion of the population aged over 65 rose from less than 10% in 1960 to 17% in 2015, and is projected to reach 28% by 2050 (OECD, 2017a). Many of these people are living with dementia. In Canada, for example, dementia prevalence in the population 65 and over reached 7.1% in 2013 (Public Health Agency of Canada, 2017). Moreover, the share of the population over 80 in the OECD is projected to increase from nearly 5% in 2015 to more than 10% by 2050 (OECD, 2017a) (Figure 1.2). As populations continue to age, the prevalence of dementia in OECD countries is also expected to rise, from an estimated 18.7 million people in 2017 to 40.9 million by 2050. The pace of population ageing has been slower in non-OECD countries, although it is expected to accelerate. In large partner countries including Brazil and China, less than 2% of the population was 80 years and over in 2015, though this share is expected to reach close to 7% in Brazil and more than 8% in China by 2050.

Figure 1.2. Trends in the share of the population aged over 80 years, 1990-2050

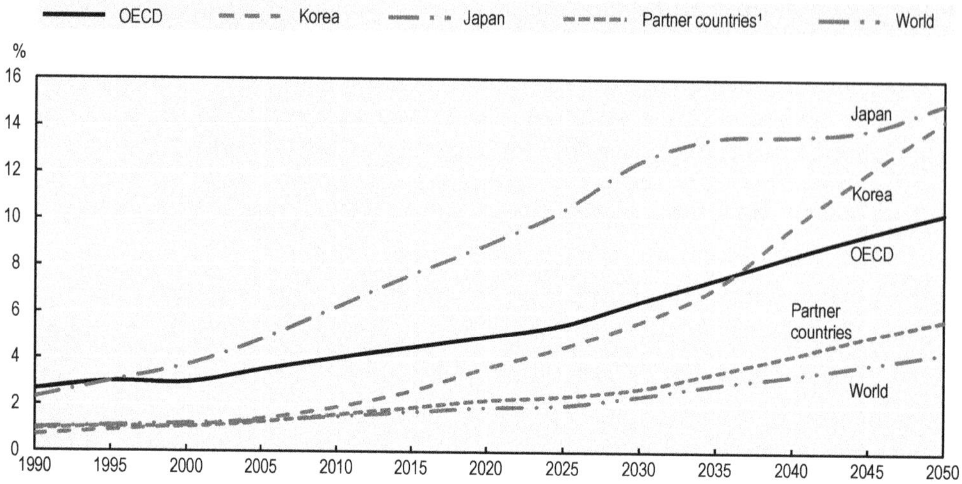

Note: Partner countries include Brazil, China, Colombia, India, Indonesia, Lithuania, Russia, Costa Rica and South Africa.
Source: OECD Historical Population Data and Projections Database, 2017.

StatLink http://dx.doi.org/10.1787/888933735044

The personal and financial costs of dementia are immense. Globally, dementia represents one of the leading causes of disability for elderly adults. It is estimated that the health and social costs of dementia reached over USD 1 trillion per year in 2018 (Alzheimer's Disease International, 2015).

Figure 1.3. Dementia prevalence

People with dementia per 1 000 population (all ages)

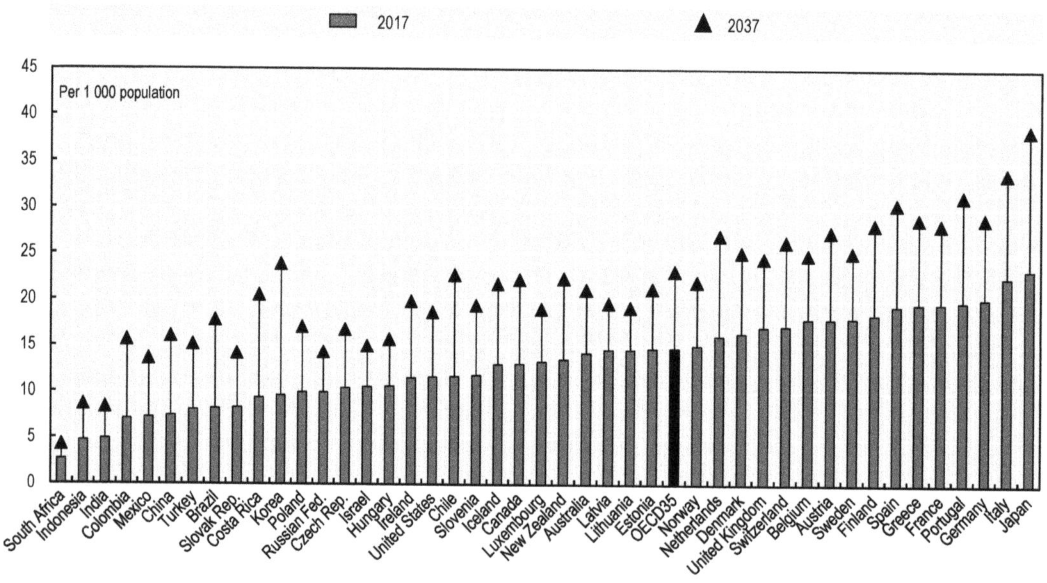

Source: *OECD Health Statistics 2017*, http://dx.doi.org/10.1787/health-data-en.

StatLink http://dx.doi.org/10.1787/888933735063

As of today, there is no cure for dementia. Even with billions of dollars spent on research and development, scientists have yet to find a cure or a disease-modifying treatment for dementia. Dementia is an extremely complex disease, and appears to take hold years or even decades before people begin to show common symptoms. This makes drug development for dementia particularly challenging, as researchers and pharmaceutical companies grapple with how to develop and test medications to be used by patients years before symptoms emerge. Promising late-stage clinical trials conducted in recent years have had disappointing results.

In the face of these challenges, attention on whether and how dementia can be prevented in the first place has grown. Some compelling evidence suggests that dementia is associated with many risk factors, including obesity, physical activity, hypertension, smoking, diabetes, hearing loss, and depression. A recent *Lancet* review suggested that up to one-third of dementia cases can likely be delayed or prevented through preventive measures (Livingston et al., 2017). The risk factors identified for dementia contribute to the development of many diseases, and broad-based prevention strategies targeting health challenges such as obesity, diabetes, or loneliness likely also affect dementia. Nevertheless, the length of time between the development of dementia and onset of symptoms makes it difficult to evaluate the effects of these preventive measures on developing dementia. The long time lag makes it problematic to evaluate, for example, the return on investment from primary prevention strategies on dementia (Livingston et al., 2017; Wittenberg et al., 2017).

A recent report by the National Academies of Science, Engineering and Medicine in the United States found that evidence related to preventive interventions is inconclusive but encouraging, and suggested making available information related to cognitive training, blood pressure management, and physical activity as interventions that may serve a protective role against cognitive decline (Leshner et al., 2017).

In recent years, some evidence has emerged to suggest that the risk of developing dementia can possibly be reduced. Recent longitudinal studies in the United States and United Kingdom (England and Wales) have found that dementia prevalence fell in recent decades (Matthews et al., 2013; Langa et al., 2017). These findings have highlighted the potential of harnessing preventive measures to attenuate the rapid increase in dementia prevalence. Nevertheless, even with declines in dementia prevalence, the rapid ageing worldwide all but guarantees significant growth in the population living with dementia in the coming decades.

In this context, health and social care services are crucial to people who develop dementia and their families. The progress of dementia cannot be stopped until a cure or disease-modifying treatment for dementia is developed. Nevertheless, the quality of life and level of cognitive impairment that people with dementia experience along the way can be much improved. Health and social care services are critical to ensuring that people who develop dementia, and their families, can enjoy a high quality of life throughout the course of their lives.

Box 1.1. Reducing the risk of cognitive impairment: Recent evidence from the FINGER study

Though the precise disease pathway of dementia disorders is not well understood, there is growing evidence to suggest that socioeconomic and lifestyle-related factors can impact the onset of symptoms including cognitive impairment. Physical activity, nutrition, social connections or loneliness, and level of education have all been associated with a risk of developing dementia.

A recent randomised control trial of older Finnish adults, the Finnish Geriatric Intervention Study to Prevent Cognitive Impairment and Disability (FINGER), indicates that risk reduction interventions can impact the development of cognitive impairment (Ngandu et al., 2015). Older adults who were randomised into the intervention group received a multi-domain intervention that included physical activity, advising on nutrition, cognitive training, and follow-up and management for metabolic and vascular risk factors (Kivipelto et al., 2013). After two years of follow-up, levels of cognitive impairment were significantly higher among the control than the intervention group.

Results from the FINGER study indicate that intervening early to reduce the lifestyle risks associated with dementia may help to maintain cognitive function and delay the onset of cognitive impairment. The promising results of the FINGER trial have led to the creation of a network of research studies that aim to replicate the findings of the FINGER study in other contexts, including the United States (US-POINTER) and Singapore (SINGER) (Kivipelto, Mangialasche, & Ngandu, 2018).

1.2. Improving diagnosis to facilitate access to treatment and care

1.2.1. Dementia remains underdiagnosed or is diagnosed too late

A diagnosis allows health professionals to guide people with dementia and their families to the services that will be most helpful to them in order to start preparing for the challenges that the disease will present as it progresses. A formal diagnosis (see Box 1.2) is often explicitly required to qualify and be reimbursed for support and services. Without a diagnosis, people with dementia may be excluded from many support services that can help them to live well in the community for as long as possible.

Box 1.2. What is a dementia diagnosis?

A "diagnosis" means different things depending on the country and health care setting. Most simply, a diagnosis of dementia means that someone is told by a health professional that, in their opinion, they have dementia. In some cases, a diagnosis of dementia enables someone to access certain health and social care services, or would make them eligible for additional reimbursement. This may require specific tests to be carried out, specialists to be consulted, or for the diagnosis to be made in a specified setting.

Promoting access to diagnosis is a priority for many OECD countries and some improvements have been seen in recent years. In the United Kingdom (England), for example, a key target of the Prime Minister's Challenge on Dementia aimed to increase the diagnosis rate to two-thirds of people estimated to have dementia. Between 2010 and 2017, the diagnosis rate in England rose from 42.6% to 67.6%.

Nonetheless, in most countries the majority of people with dementia have not been diagnosed. In Denmark, for example, the number of people registered with a diagnosis in the national patient registry represents 43.6% of the total number estimated to have dementia. Even those who have been diagnosed may have been identified too late to get benefit from care and the few available treatments. For example, medications such as memantine, donepezil and rivastigmine can help improve cognition and behaviour for certain forms of mild to moderate dementias. Advance care planning allows people with dementia to outline their preferences for care before they develop serious cognitive difficulties, and is in many cases legally binding. If initiated in time, advance care planning can help people with dementia ensure their care follows their wishes, even after they are no longer able to communicate their needs.

1.2.2. Primary care doctors play a key role in dementia diagnosis, but lack support and competences to do so

In 26 OECD countries, primary care doctors act as the first point of contact and can carry out initial testing and provide an indicative diagnosis before referring people on to specialists as necessary (see Table 1.1).

Table 1.1. Dementia diagnosis and care roles carried out by primary care physicians

	First point of contact	Indicative diagnosis	Formal diagnosis	Initiating medications
Australia	X	X	X	X
Austria	X	X		
Belgium	X	X		
Canada (British Columbia)	X	X	X	X
Chile	X	X	X	X
Czech Republic	X	X		
Denmark	X	X	X	
Estonia	X			
Finland	X	X		
France	X	X		
Germany	X	X		
Greece		X		
Hungary	X			
Ireland	X	X		
Israel	X	X		
Luxembourg	X	X		
Mexico	X	X		
Netherlands	X	X	X	X
New Zealand	X	X	X	X
Norway	X	X	X	X
Portugal	X	X		
Slovak Republic	X	X		
Slovenia	X	X		
Sweden	X	X	X	X
Switzerland	X	X	X	X
Turkey				
United Kingdom (England)	X	X	In some cases (rare)	
United States	X	X		

Source: OECD Dementia Care Policy Interviews 2017.

However, many primary care doctors lack the skills and experience needed to make an effective diagnosis. Some primary care doctors report that they are not confident or comfortable diagnosing dementia and there is evidence that diagnostic outcomes are poor. A survey of general practitioners in Denmark suggested that less than half of primary care practitioners were able to perform a good assessment of dementia (Waldorff and Moller, 2001, Waldorff et al., 2003). Other studies have found that primary care doctors correctly identify only around 75% of dementia cases, and often fail to record the diagnoses they make. The performance of primary care is worse with more complex cases, such as early-stage cognitive impairment (Mitchell et al., 2011).

While primary care doctors should and usually do play a central role in dementia diagnosis, they need the skills and resources to do this job well. One way countries can do this is to develop clinical guidelines to support primary care doctors in making better diagnoses. Such guidelines already exist in at least 16 OECD countries, including Australia, Canada, Chile, Denmark, New Zealand, Sweden, and the United Kingdom, either in the form of dementia-specific guidelines or as broader guidelines that cover dementia and other health conditions. Where guidelines do not exist, countries should consider developing them. However, even where guidelines exist, there is evidence that practice regularly diverges from them. Even after primary care physicians were made aware of clinical guidelines for dementia care in Denmark, for example, no difference was found in how doctors actually practiced.

More may also need to be done to raise awareness of guidelines among doctors and to give them the skills to apply them. In particular, dementia training for primary care doctors is essential for high-quality diagnosis and management. While primary care doctors in all OECD countries receive some dementia training in medical school, this can be limited to a few hours in total. Although continuing education programme on dementia are available at least in 17 OECD countries, the participation rate can be low. No country requires physicians to take dementia training as part of continuing education requirements. Policy-makers need to remove barriers and promote take-up of these training courses among primary care doctors.

More national-level training courses are needed to address geographical variations in availability. Many courses are currently offered locally by non-governmental organisations, which lead to geographical variations in access. More countries could consider developing nationally available courses. In Australia, for example, a nationwide training programme, Dementia Training Australia, has made available dementia care development training opportunities for professional upskilling, and access to accredited dementia care training courses across the country

Removing barriers or providing incentives can increase take-up of dementia training. Primary care doctors may lose income if they attend a training course on dementia, so countries should consider steps to ensure that training courses are offered as part of continuous development programmes that doctors are required to undertake, or that such trainings are reimbursed. In Denmark, for example, physicians are reimbursed for the time taken away from their practice spent in training. Other countries have developed non-financial incentives with a view to increasing take-up rates. The Karolinska Institute in Sweden, for example, offers a Master's Degree in Dementia Care for Physicians, which confers greater professional recognition to dementia training. However, such schemes remain rare. Countries should assess the barriers to take-up of dementia training among primary care doctors, and consider how they can be reduced. They should also consider providing financial or non-financial incentives to boost participation.

1.2.3. People with dementia should receive an appropriate, timely diagnosis that allows them to access available care and support

Receiving a specific diagnosis can be important for identifying the best available care and treatment. However, in most cases, a full diagnose of dementia still requires advanced diagnostic tools, such as a CT scan or MRI, that are expensive to administer. Moreover, receiving a firm diagnosis requires consultation with specialists, including neurologists and psychiatrists, who are more experienced in dementia care. All of this, in a context where a cure or dementia modifying treatment is still unviable, raises questions about how best to balance the relative costs and benefits of these services.

Memory clinics – clinical settings where health professionals (often specialists) provide advanced diagnostic services – have received growing attention for their role in both diagnosis and management. Though specialists can operate independently, memory clinics have increasingly emerged as an important step in the dementia care pathway.

Box 1.3. What is a memory clinic?

Despite the rising profile of memory clinics in dementia care, what a memory clinic is has different interpretations in different settings. Originally, memory clinics served as specialised clinical settings where health professionals – often neurologists, geriatricians, or psychiatrists – provided advanced diagnostic services.

In this report, we define memory clinics most broadly as any clinical setting where health professionals provide advanced diagnostic services and define themselves, or are defined externally, as memory clinics. More specifically, we consider clinics that provide diagnostic services but no or only limited follow-up care to be diagnostic memory clinics. Memory clinics that are integrated into defined care pathways or otherwise engage in care management, education or training, and other components of dementia care are defined here as comprehensive memory clinics.

At least 25 OECD countries have developed memory clinics (Box 1.3). Memory clinics have also expanded rapidly in recent years. The number of memory clinics doubled in the United Kingdom between 1993 and 2000 and quadrupled in New Zealand between 2003 and 2008. The number of people aged 65 years and over per memory clinic varies seven-fold across countries, from more than 170 000 people 65 and over per memory clinic in Belgium to about 23 000 per memory clinic in France. While the concentration of memory clinics within countries also differs, this national variation indicates that different countries rely to different extents on memory clinics as a part of the clinical pathway for dementia.

In recent years, memory clinics in some countries expanded their services beyond diagnostic testing to include follow-up care and support for people living with dementia and even family members. However, the effectiveness – and particularly cost-effectiveness – of diagnosis and care through a memory clinic is not clear. A recent study of memory assessment services in the United Kingdom found that while the care provided through memory clinics was effective, it was not cost-effective (Gomes et al., 2017). A randomised control trial of follow-up care through memory clinics in the Netherlands found that care provided through memory clinics was no more effective than post-diagnostic support provided through general practitioners (Meeuwsen et al., 2012). Given the cost pressures faced by many health and social care systems, there is a need for better understanding under what conditions memory clinics can add best value to other dementia care services, and countries should also carefully consider the appropriateness of memory clinics in the clinical pathway, particularly for post-diagnostic support.

There is still a long way to go to improve the process of diagnosis. Specialist memory clinic services continue to play an important role in diagnosis, but their role should be better defined. Just five countries in the OECD (Denmark, France, the Netherlands, Switzerland and the United Kingdom) have developed or are developing definitions, guidelines and standards for memory clinics. This means that the care provided can differ significantly from one clinic to the next, even within the same region of a country.

1.2.4. Dementia remains difficult to identify and measure.

Dementia has been a policy priority for many countries in recent years. At least 22 OECD countries have developed national plans or strategies to improve their country's dementia response, and many have launched policies aimed at improving management and care. However, data on dementia remains extremely limited, and can hamper efforts to identify people living with dementia. Without better identification of who has dementia, it remains challenging to improve quality of care and outcomes.

Improving data for dementia is recognised as a key policy in a number of national action and strategic plans, including in Ireland, Switzerland, the United Kingdom, and the United States. Other countries have made improving dementia research — not only clinical research, but also population health — a key component of their national plans, including Australia, Finland, and Mexico. Yet despite these signals, few countries have data systems that can generate the kind of information critical to developing evidence-based policies and measuring progress toward defined goals. Data challenges have further constrained the ability to engage in international comparisons in addition to hampering effective domestic policy development. Though most countries can estimate dementia prevalence, for example, very few have an accurate estimate of diagnosis rates in their country. Despite the policy focus on improving diagnosis, a recent OECD pilot data collection on dementia care indicators found that fewer than 40% of countries could estimate diagnosis rates on a national level (Figure 1.4). An accurate picture of the number of people living with, developing, and being diagnosed with dementia is critical in order to understand the effect of new policies.

Figure 1.4. Countries able to measure different aspects of dementia care

Out of 21 OECD countries

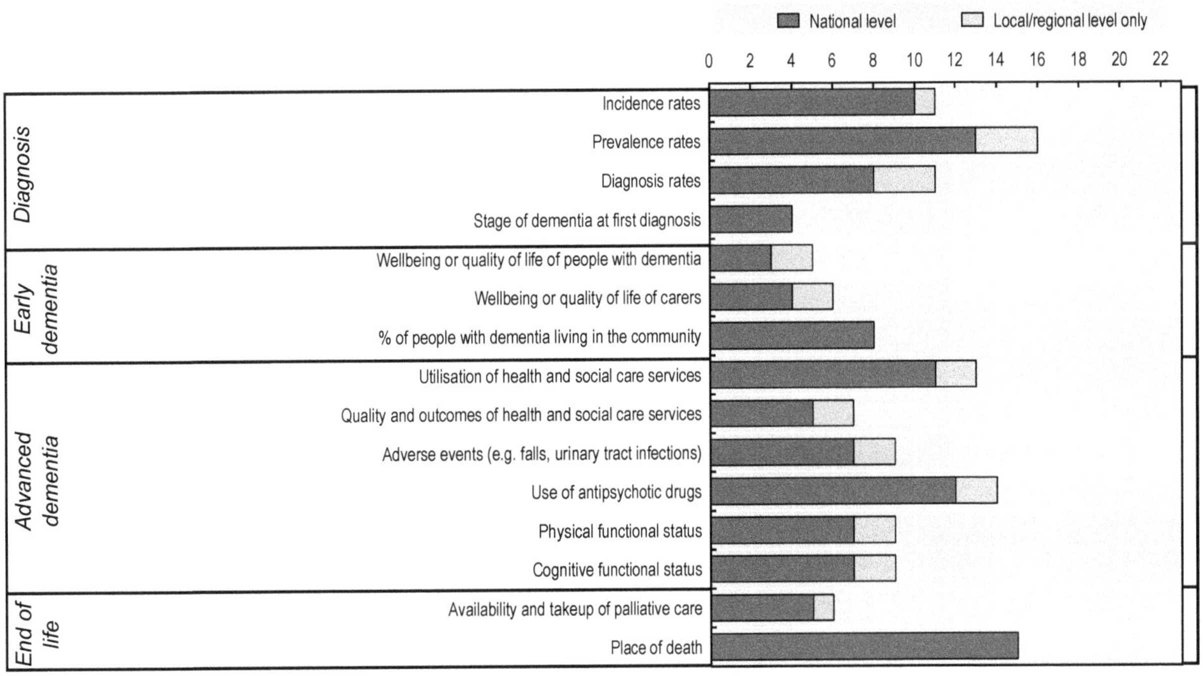

Source: OECD Dementia Care Quality Feasibility Study 2016.

StatLink http://dx.doi.org/10.1787/888933735082

Countries across the OECD have developed a range of processes to collect, store, share, link, protect and use health data. They are at very different stages when it comes to how advanced and widespread these data systems are. These different approaches can have real implications for how health services are delivered and diseases are managed and monitored. Where diagnoses are made in primary and secondary care, for example, data from just secondary care would provide an insufficient estimate of the rate of diagnosis and the number of people who receive health services for dementia. Connecting the information collected across health care settings can therefore give a better picture of the real state of health system quality. This is particularly important for dementia, where primary care plays a major role in diagnosis and care management. Yet less than half of countries reported that they could identify people with dementia from primary care records on a national level (Figure 1.5).

Figure 1.5. Countries that can identify people with dementia in administrative data

By care setting (out of 21 OECD countries)

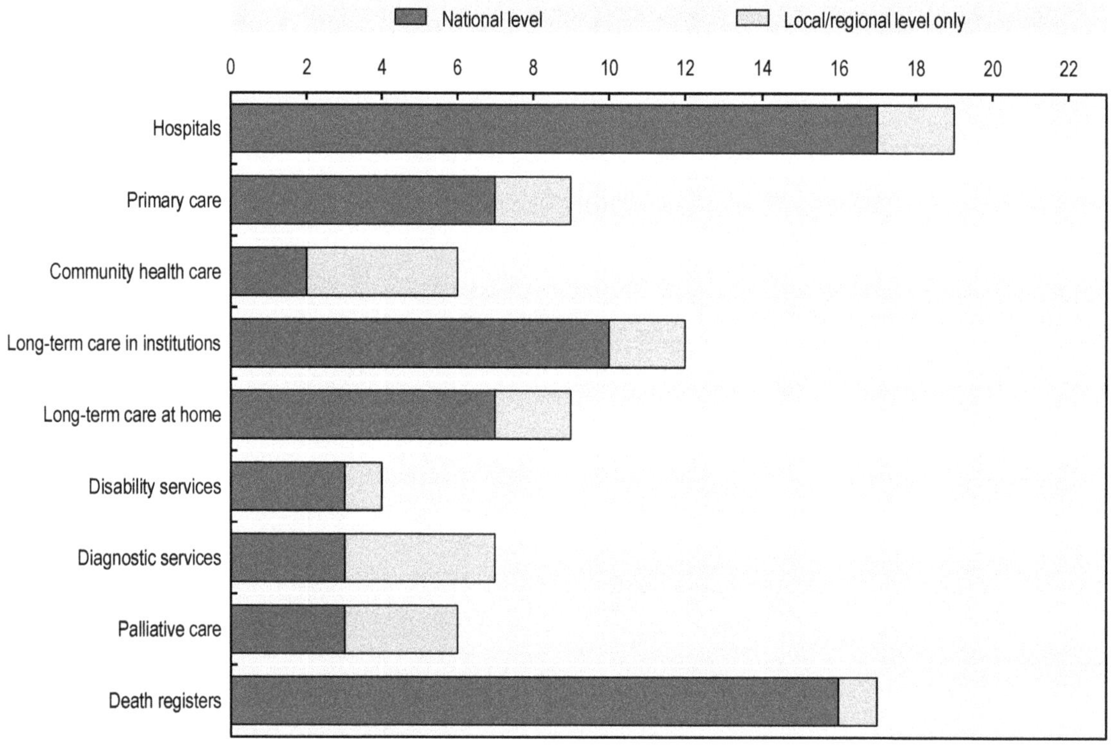

Source: OECD Dementia Care Quality Feasibility Study 2016.

StatLink http://dx.doi.org/10.1787/888933735101

A number of OECD countries have aimed to improve the data landscape by linking data from a number of national datasets. Slightly over half of countries surveyed for *Health Data Governance: Privacy, Monitoring and Research* reported that they regularly linked data from at least four large national datasets (OECD, 2015b). Countries frequently link data from hospital inpatient datasets, mortality data, cancer registries, prescriptions registries, and census databases. However, even with these data sources linked, important areas of the health system are frequently excluded from regular data linking. This is particularly problematic for monitoring the quality of care and outcomes for dementia. Many of the less frequently linked data sets come from areas of the health system, such as primary care, that come into frequent contact with people with dementia, and long-term care.

Given its important and growing role, primary care is a crucial data source to ensure that individual patients receive the best quality care they can. The role of primary care for dementia has increased in many OECD countries. Yet primary care data systems are often separated from broader health data systems, with very few countries linking primary care data to other sources of health data. Less than 10% of surveyed OECD countries reported regularly linking data from primary care with other health records to monitor quality and performance (OECD, 2015b). This can have serious implications for how health professionals respond to patients with dementia. For example, patients managed and diagnosed in primary care may not have their diagnosis communicated in case of a hospital admission, which may affect how they are treated during their stay. Moreover, primary care physicians may not have the incentive to fully record information related to the dementia diagnosis in their medical records. During the development of the dementia disease registry in Sweden, primary care physicians were initially given financial incentives to record assessments in the registry. Moreover, even where physicians may wish to record dementia, coding practices can be complex and they may lack the guidance or training to do so accurately. In the United Kingdom (England), a survey of coding practices among general practitioners in London found that a basic coding exercise that helped practitioners recode cases of dementia increased the number of people recorded to have a diagnosis of dementia by nearly 9% (Russell et al., 2013). Guidance documents developed by NHS England in London and the North Region aim to improve the accuracy of dementia coding in primary care.

A number of countries have adopted the registry model to monitor and improve outcomes for people living with dementia. The registry model has been used regularly to monitor other diseases, such as cancer, and can help to increase data transparency and contribute to better outcomes, often at a lower cost of care. In recent years, some countries have applied the disease registry model to dementia. While the depth and coverage differs between countries, the development of registries reflects an effort to improve data quality and transparency around dementia.

Six OECD countries –Denmark, France, Israel, Norway, Sweden and the United States – have developed dementia registries at either the national or regional level. In Sweden, for example, the Swedish Dementia Registry *SveDem* collects information from all memory clinics, nearly 80% of general practices, and long-term care settings. In addition to demographic and clinical indicators, information on non-pharmacological treatments, community-based support, quality of life, and other measures provides a more comprehensive picture of how someone with dementia is living with the disease. In addition to *SveDem*, Sweden has additionally developed a Behavioural and Psychological Symptoms of Dementia (BPSD) registry that aims to improve quality of care in nursing homes.

1.3. People with dementia struggle to live independently because initiatives to make communities safe, accessible and socially inclusive remain fragmented

1.3.1. Ageing at home reflects both the preferences of people with dementia and government priorities, but community-based care is not fit for purpose

OECD countries have begun to encourage ageing at home for as long as possible, and the number of beds in long-term care facilities has fallen across the OECD (Figure 1.6). This corresponds to the preferences of many older people, including those with dementia. Maintaining relationships and social connections are particularly important for people living with dementia, because loneliness and isolation can accelerate the progression of the disease. By living at home, people with dementia are better able to stay independent through the early stages of the condition and connected to their communities. Community-based interventions are often also more cost-effective for health systems, and can deliver a higher quality of life, at least until a certain level of disability.

Figure 1.6. Trends in long-term beds in institutions and hospitals, 2005-15

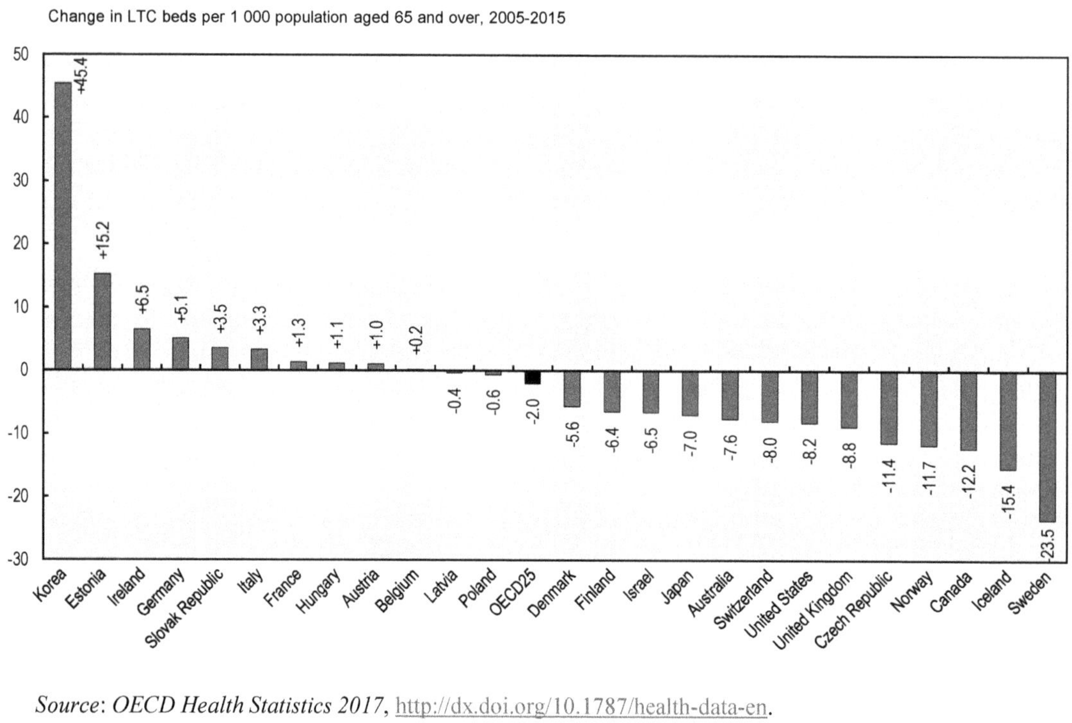

Source: *OECD Health Statistics 2017*, http://dx.doi.org/10.1787/health-data-en.

StatLink http://dx.doi.org/10.1787/888933735120

Living at home with dementia can, however, pose unique challenges as the disease progresses and symptoms, such as wandering, increase. Once-familiar home environments can become difficult and even hazardous to navigate, and can contribute to accidents, such as falls. Assistive technologies, such as location tracking devices and automatic reminders, can help people with daily activities, though uptake is not always high. Moreover, community services and activities may be underprepared to accommodate people living with dementia.

1.3.2. Better care co-ordination is important for people with dementia, especially those with complex needs.

Many health and social care services have been developed to help slow cognitive decline and improve quality of life for people with dementia and their families. Cognitive stimulation therapy has been found in some cases to help improve memory as well as available medications (Knapp et al., 2006; Spector et al., 2003). Moreover, even services that do not improve memory can have positive impacts on the well-being of people with dementia and their families. Exercise therapies can help to improve functional ability, for example, while arts- and music-based therapies can help to reduce behavioural and emotional symptoms (Cowl & Gaugler, 2014). But navigating these services remains difficult. Many people do not know what services are available to them, or how to access them. Non-medical therapies are often delivered by non-governmental services, such as local Alzheimer's Associations, that are outside of health and long-term care benefit packages. Waiting lists to access services can also be long. In Greece, for example, demand to attend day care centres far exceeds the approximately 5000 places available.

In this context, coordinated post-diagnostic support, for example through established care co-ordination pathways or case managers, can help people obtain the best support they can and access disparate services in a systematic manner. Post-diagnostic care pathways have been developed specifically for people living with dementia in at least nine countries. In Scotland, for example, the government mandated that all people diagnosed with dementia receive one year of post-diagnostic support, and created 'dementia link workers' to help people access what is available to them. In Norway, municipal memory teams provide both pre- and post-diagnostic support to people diagnosed with dementia. The memory teams are distinct from Norway's more general care co-ordination, which is available to any individuals requiring services from more than one health or social care agency. Similar models of coordinated, dementia-specific care have been developed in other countries. Without dedicated support, post-diagnostic care may be left up to the diagnosing physicians, who may not see many cases of dementia and may not be familiar with the services that would be available to them.

People with complex cases of dementia in particular may benefit from targeted post-diagnostic support. Early onset dementia or minority cultural and language backgrounds also pose additional barriers to accessing services, which tend to be designed for a typical patient profile. Some countries have therefore developed case management programmes that are available to complex or rare cases. The Maisons pour l'Autonomie et l'Intégration des Maladies Alzheimer (MAIA) in France, for example, offers a single entry point to health and long-term care for very complex cases. In Estonia, people with early onset dementia are eligible for a separate system of support, provided through the National Insurance Board. Qualifying patients receive state care services, including individual case management services and personalised rehabilitation plans. While the programme is not limited to those with dementia (among others, people with schizophrenia and other psychiatric conditions are also eligible), special care services only support people with dementia under the age of 65, after which they must use the services available in their local municipality.

Special case management programmes for people with early onset dementia are similarly available in Australia, where the National Younger Onset Dementia Key Worker Program, funded by the Department of Social Services, provides case management support to people under the age of 65. People with symptoms of dementia who have not yet been diagnosed are also eligible for support through the Dementia Key Worker Program, where case managers can help people receive a formal diagnosis. In Norway, clinical care guidelines have developed a separate care pathway for people with early-onset dementia, complex cases, and cases that involve people from minority language and cultural backgrounds.

1.3.3. Strengthening community services would reduce health risks and social isolation and improve integration for people with dementia

While ageing at home often aligns with the wishes of older people, including those with dementia, people with dementia can often face challenges that make staying in the community particularly difficult. Communities are often inadequately prepared, including dealing with problems related to unintentional wandering, challenges with driving and using public transportation, lack of understanding from people in the community and the service industry, and exploitation, such as elder abuse and fraud. Developing interventions that can help reduce the risks that people with dementia may face in the community is important to enabling a high quality of life.

Dementia-friendly initiatives that reduce stigma and improve community response have been effective. Community members are well-placed to look out for possible dementia symptoms amongst their peers. In recent years, nearly all OECD countries have developed 'dementia-friendly' community initiatives that aim to improve awareness and reduce the stigma associated with the disease, thereby helping to build more inclusive societies. They increase general awareness, take into account the needs of people with dementia when planning and designing services, and improve the local business and general community response. Such initiatives have been well received by both dementia advocates and local communities. In the United Kingdom and Japan, training the public to become dementia friends has been extremely successful. More than two million 'dementia friends' have trained in England, while more than 9.5 million people have attended training sessions to become so-called 'dementia supporters' in Japan.

Another possibility to strengthen local services is by engaging local businesses and public services, as a way to improve the daily experience for the many people living at home with dementia. Some countries have developed programmes to improve the response of public services and local businesses to people living with dementia. A training programme in Austria that teaches police officers de-escalation approaches to help respond to people exhibiting behavioural and psychological symptoms of dementia (BPSD) has trained at least 2 000 police officers since it was started in 2013.

In another example, at least five OECD countries – Australia, Belgium (Flanders), Canada, the United Kingdom, the United States – have launched training programmes for local pharmacists. As trusted health professionals who are often in frequent contact with their older patients, pharmacists are well-placed to monitor behavioural changes and provide advice and signposting for people who need help. In Flanders, Belgium, for example, the Flemish Pharmacist Network has worked with the Flemish Dementia Expertise Centre to increase the role of pharmacists, together with primary care practitioners, in supporting people with dementia. The programme aims to train pharmacists throughout Flanders to ensure they have the necessary knowledge and information to both identify the first signs of dementia and provide information and support, including referrals on to further services, to people living with dementia and their family members. Programmes like these serve a double purpose. They can both improve the quality of services given to people with dementia, and improve understanding for dementia among people who may not have regular opportunities to learn about the disease. In doing so, they make living in the community both easier and more welcoming for people with dementia.

Health and social care professionals who are trained in dementia care and familiar with local services should be available in local communities, too. The services available to support people with dementia can vary substantially by community. People living with dementia and their families already face a range of challenges that make coordinating these services difficult.

At least four countries – Chile, Denmark, Finland and Norway – have developed new professional staff positions and resource centres that are focused on supporting people with dementia who live in the community. Community-based dementia staff positions have in some cases become the first point of contact for people with dementia or their carers, sometimes before a formal diagnosis has even been made. In Norway, for example, 'memory teams' operate in 75% of municipalities and provide both pre-diagnostic support and follow-up assistance to people with dementia and their families. In Chile, 'community managers' help to identify and follow-up with people who live with dementia in the community and provide a relatable source of support and information to them. In Denmark, most municipalities have dementia co-ordinators who perform similar functions, visiting people concerned about dementia symptoms prior to a diagnostic evaluation, and offering help in coordinating care after a diagnosis is made. A network of memory nurses across Finland, located in primary health care clinics, perform similar counselling and coordinating functions for people with dementia and their families, particularly those with advanced forms of the disease who live in the community. These positions can work together with or alongside existing care co-ordination and case management systems. Community-based guidance staff can help people not only navigate the logistics of their care, but also learn to live with dementia in the best way they can.

1.3.4. There is little standardised measurement of outcomes for people living with dementia

Despite the strong policy emphasis on improving community-based care for people living with dementia, measurement is lagging in most countries. Few countries regularly measure the proportion of people with dementia living in the community: Eight of 21 OECD countries can estimate the proportion of people with dementia living in the community, while 11 out of 21 OECD countries can identify those with a diagnosis who receive home-based long-term care services.

Clear outcome goals for dementia-friendly initiatives are often missing, or are focused on intermediate outcomes such as the number of dementia-friendly communities or volunteers trained. Given the focus of many dementia care policies on improving quality of life, countries should consider how to better capture person-centred indicators including self-reported quality of life measures for people with dementia and their carers. Quality of life measures offer a good opportunity to measure whether community-based initiatives, which usually focus on well-being more than clinical outcomes, are working. While most community-based interventions are focused on improving autonomy and quality of life, measurement of quality of life is notably lacking from regular data collection in almost all OECD countries. Two countries – Australia and Canada – are able to measure wellbeing or quality of life for people with dementia nationally and on a regular basis.

1.4. Informal carers are the most important source of support for many people with dementia, but not enough support is available to them.

1.4.1. Informal carers provide a majority of dementia care, but caring for a person with dementia is mentally and physically taxing

Family and friends play a critical role in caring for people with dementia. Dementia affects not just the people who receive a diagnosis, but can also be devastating for the families and loved ones around them. Family members and friends often provide care, either on top of or in place of the support offered through formal care systems. Informal care is estimated to represent 40% of the total cost of dementia worldwide. It can be substantially more where formal care services are less well established. As people live at home longer, and the burden of dementia rises, the need for family members and others to provide additional care will continue to rise.

Figure 1.7. Share of informal carers among population aged 50 and over,
2015 (or nearest year)

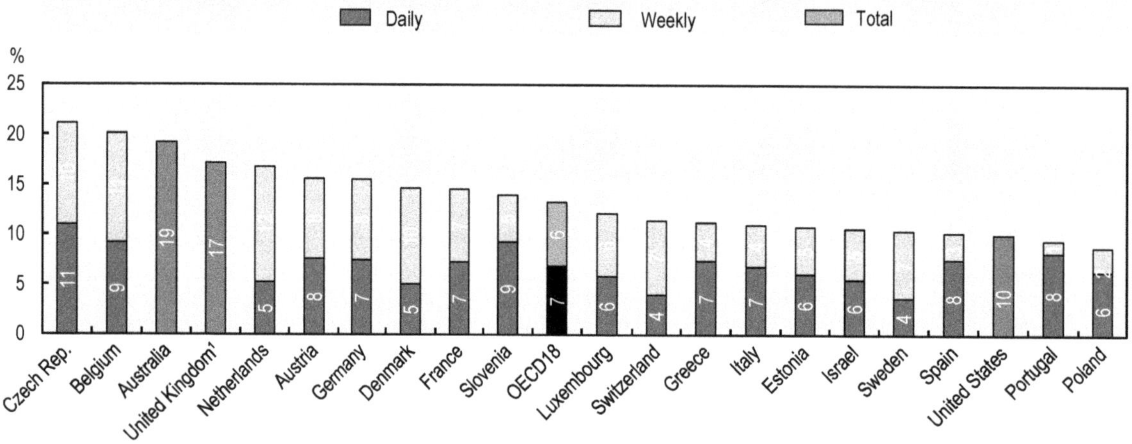

Note: United Kingdom refers to England. The definition of informal carers differs between surveys.
Source: OECD Health Statistics 2017, http://dx.doi.org/10.1787/health-data-en.

StatLink http://dx.doi.org/10.1787/888933735139

The difficult behavioural and psychological challenges that can arise from dementia, and the emotional strain of caring for someone with memory loss, can place a high burden on carers and lead to burn-out, depression, anxiety, and poor physical health. A longitudinal study using data from the United States found that women who provided intensive caregiving (36 hours or more per week) to a spouse were nearly six times more likely to be depressed or anxious (Cannuscio et al., 2002). Caregivers are much more likely to report a poorer quality of life than similar adults who do not care for family or friends (Thomas et al., 2015; Stansfeld et al., 2014; Pinquart & Sörensen, 2003). Notably, caregivers supporting people living with dementia are much more likely to experience poorer mental and physical health than non-carers and non-dementia caregivers (Stansfeld et al., 2014; Pinquart & Sörensen, 2003; Ory et al., 1999). High caregiver stress can also increase the chance that the person they care for will be put in a long-term care facility, and can increase the behavioural and psychological symptoms of dementia.

1.4.2. Most caregiver policies are not tailored to the needs of caring for people with dementia.

Countries recognise the important role that informal care plays to support people with long-term conditions, and have taken steps to ensure that caring for a loved one does not come at the expense of the carer's own well-being. However, most carer support interventions have been designed for informal carers more broadly, and do not necessarily focus on carers of people with dementia, or reflect the unique needs of dementia carers. The length of time many informal carers will spend supporting a person with dementia, as well as the high stress of the role, means that caregivers of people with dementia may sometimes have unique needs that broad-based policies may not necessarily meet.

Employment policies should be supportive and flexible for caregivers in the workforce. For informal carers who are in the workforce, juggling the responsibilities of a job and caregiver can cause considerable stress, and impact how well a carer can perform their duties. Improving caregiver health is also important to the well-being of those they care for.

Caregiver burden is an important determinant of early institutionalization (D'Onofrio et al., 2014; Gallagher et al., 2011; Mittelman et al., 2006; Gaugler et al., 2009; Spillman and Long, 2009; Yaffe et al., 2002). Multiple studies suggest that higher caregiver stress increases the desire and likelihood to institutionalise care recipients with dementia. Beyond the broad category of "caregiver stress," financial difficulty, physical stress, social support, family cohesion and caregiver knowledge about dementia have been associated with higher desire and risk of institutionalisation (Gallagher et al., 2011; Spitznagel et al., 2006; Spillman and Long, 2009). Caregiver burden is particularly high when people with dementia have high needs, including exhibiting the behavioural and psychological symptoms of dementia (BPSD) (Vaingankar et al., 2016).

Caregiver burden and health have also been associated with worse health outcomes for their recipients of care. Caregivers of people with dementia with higher levels of burden, caring intensity, depression, and lower educational attainment have been found to report higher levels of behavioural and psychiatric symptoms of dementia (BPSD) among care recipients (Sink et al., 2006). Higher caregiver burden has also been associated with a higher prevalence of falls among care recipients (Vaughon et al., 2018; Kuzuya et al., 2006).

Researchers have suggested promoting interventions that reduce these and other sources of caregiver stress as a means of delaying institutionalisation and improving health outcomes among people with dementia. As of 2017, 27 of the 35 OECD countries have workplace support policies in place that allow informal carers to take at least some time off to provide care. In 19 countries, at least some part of the time off is offered as paid leave, though this tends to be very short. However, the length of time many informal carers will spend supporting a person with dementia, as well as the high stress of doing so, means that these provisions are often insufficient.

1.4.3. Day care services and training should be strengthened and better signposted

Respite care, which offers carers the opportunity to take a short break away from caring, can help caregivers to make space to focus on their own needs. Day care services can allow carers to attend to other activities on a regular basis, while overnight respite care can help to facilitate longer-term breaks and allows caregivers to recharge from the daily stresses of their role. While further research is needed, day care respite services have been found likely to be cost-effective (Knapp, Iemmi and Romeo, 2013). Nearly all countries have some form of day care available, though uptake can depend on the quality and accessibility of local services. Programmes that can work around the needs of carers – for example, those that offer pick-up and drop-off services, or schedule day care hours to fit around the schedules of caregivers who work – can contribute to making day care services work for both the person with dementia and their carer. In Switzerland, for example, day care centres in Lucerne have begun offering full-service support around the day care activities. Staff members come to the person's home to help them get ready for the day before driving them to and from day care. Overnight respite care is more dependent on local capacity constraints, and many people who could benefit from the service are not able to access it.

People who care for friends or family members with dementia will almost always benefit from training or skill-building support to help them in their new role. Training and support programmes are widely available for caregivers of people with dementia, and are most often delivered through the non-governmental sector, such as through local branches of the Alzheimer's Association. In the United States, the Resources for Enhancing Alzheimer's Caregiving Health (REACH) intervention was implemented across the Department of Veterans Affairs (Nichols et al., 2011, Nichols et al., 2017). Where services are not delivered through the health or social care sectors, it is important that health professionals are familiar with the services offered through non-governmental organisations. This will help to ensure that people receive the support they need, irrespective of how it is delivered.

Signposting carers to support should be made a standard part of the post-diagnostic care pathway. In addition to the general carer programmes available, many services for dementia carers are offered through non-governmental organisations and locally-based services. However, it may not be clear to the carer what services are available and what support is beneficial. Information about and referrals to available services for carers should be consistently integrated into post-diagnostic care. An example of effective co-ordination between the clinical setting and support services can be found in the United States, at the Healthy Aging Brain Centre in Indiana. Both people with dementia and their caregivers undergo a needs assessment, and staff members are trained to evaluate the level of burden on the caregiver and refer them to support services available in the community.

1.5. Care for people with advanced dementia lacks dignity and can result in worse health outcomes

1.5.1. Most residential homes are not designed to address the needs of people with dementia, while smaller scale housing shows promising results

Even with good community-based care, some people with dementia will eventually develop care needs that cannot necessarily be supported at home, and will require more intensive facility-based support. Long-term care facilities such as nursing homes must therefore be equipped to provide high-quality, person-centred support for people with dementia. A majority of nursing home residents have cognitive impairment and dementia, though many of them have not been diagnosed. Studies in Europe (Czech Republic, England, Finland, France, Germany, Israel, Italy, Netherlands, Sweden) indicate that close to 70% of nursing home residents have some form of cognitive impairment (Onder et al., 2012; Björk et al., 2016). Yet traditional models of long-term care living may not be suitable for people with dementia. The physical design of many residences, such as long hallways, locked wards, and hospital-like facilities can contribute to confusion and distress among residents, and nursing homes are frequently under-resourced and understaffed, which can contribute to care decisions that may not be in the best interest of the resident.

Small-scale units can promote social engagement and community interaction. In recent years, a number of innovative residential care models have emerged that reflect an alternative model of long-term care living. In the Netherlands, the dementia village model allows people with dementia to enjoy a level of autonomy inaccessible to most people living in care facilities, by developing an entire community of care centred around the needs of people with dementia.

New approaches to residential care share a similar emphasis on promoting smaller-scale housing that encourages community engagement and independence. Small-scale living communities, in which a small number of residents share a home and care support, can provide high-quality care and promote autonomy and a sense of community well into the advanced stages of dementia.

Multi-generational communities that accommodate both elderly populations, including those with dementia, and younger populations such as students have emerged as an approach to combat social isolation. This approach, which is in place in some care facilities in the Netherlands, United States, and Finland, offers free or reduced rent for students in exchange for spending time with older residents of the facility. In Germany, the Federal Ministry for Family Affairs, Senior Citizens, Women and Youth has promoted the development of *Mehrgenerationenhäuser*, or "multi-generational housing," in people of all ages, including families with small children, live together and create a community of support and exchange. As of 2017, about 550 *Mehrgenerationenhäuser* have been developed across the country. To promote the programme, subsidies of up to EUR 40 000 (co-financed by the federal government and local municipality) are available to develop multi-generational homes.

Dementia-friendly design should be considered for new construction and building adaptation. While attention to better long-term care for people with dementia has grown, the majority of those in long-term care facilities continue to reside in residences that do not necessarily reflect best practice. A number of countries, including Denmark, Ireland, Norway, and the United Kingdom, have put in place guidelines for dementia-friendly design that lay out principles to help develop or adapt buildings and homes with the needs of people with dementia in mind. These guidelines can help to ensure that residential facilities developed today reflect new models of dementia care. In Norway, for example, residential and nursing homes built with funding from the National Bank of Housing are now required to conform to dementia-friendly design principles.

1.5.2. The quality of long-term care for people with advanced dementia is often poor

Many people develop behavioural and psychological symptoms of dementia (BPSD) as the disease progresses. These symptoms, which can include aggression, agitation, and delusions, can be highly distressing to experience and respond to. A range of non-pharmaceutical approaches have been developed to respond to BPSD. With effective management of BPSD, people with dementia can be kept comfortable and safe, and the distress of these symptoms for caregivers can be reduced. However, it can be stressful to respond to challenging behaviours and restraints continue to be used to subdue people with BPSD.

Restraints, which can include both physical restraints and antipsychotic medications, can increase health risks, restrict autonomy and do not reflect a person-centred care approach focused on improving well-being for people living with dementia. There is widespread clinical agreement that antipsychotic medications should not be used to manage most difficult behaviour. Yet rates of antipsychotic prescribing vary by a factor of more than two across OECD countries, from 30 in every 1 000 people aged 65 and over in Sweden and the Netherlands to more than 70 in Belgium and Slovenia. Such a wide variation suggests that much more needs to be done to ensure a person-centred approach to dementia care.

Figure 1.8. Antipsychotic prescribing rates across OECD countries

Per 1000 people aged 65 and over

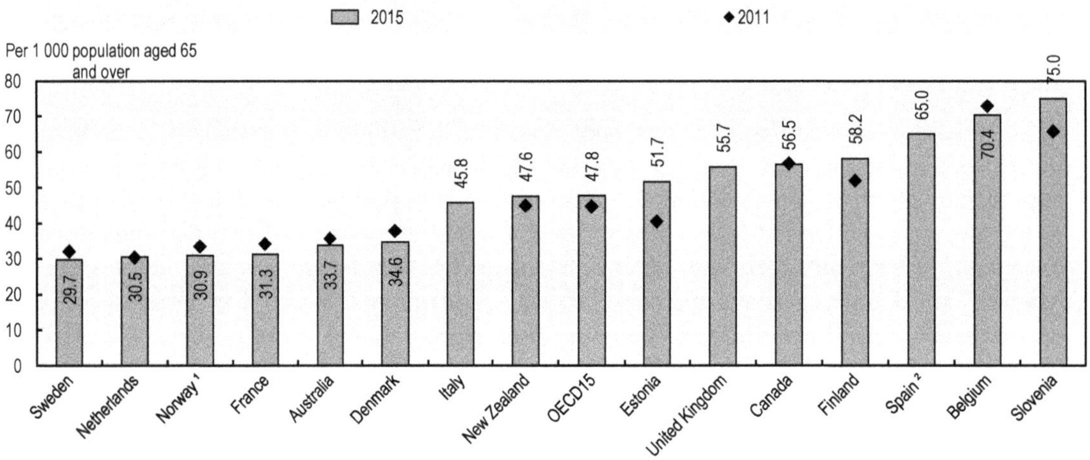

1. Data for Norway do not include people in institutional care, so underestimate the use of antipsychotics.
2. Data for Spain refer to 2014.
Source: *OECD Health Statistics 2017*, http://dx.doi.org/10.1787/health-data-en.

StatLink http://dx.doi.org/10.1787/888933735158

Guidelines and training on BPSD management are crucial to reducing inappropriate care. BPSD can be hard to manage, and adequate training and guidelines are important to ensure caregivers respond effectively to difficult situations. Guidelines and regulations around the use of physical and medical restraints can infuence how care workers and long-term care facilities respond to challenging behaviour. Financial incentives, such as requirements that long-term care facilities which receive public funding comply with directives, can help to influence behaviour. Training in restraint alternatives can increase compliance with guidelines and good practice. Staff members who have more training and work experience have a more positive outlook when confronted with difficult behaviours. In Norway, the ABC dementia training programme has helped to improve knowledge about dementia and job satisfaction. Over 19 000 basic care staff have completed the programme, with similar programmes implemented in Denmark and Sweden.

Staff who work in formal care systems – for example, care workers who are paid to work in nursing homes or as home health aides – must be adequately prepared to care for people with dementia, who often have more complex needs than other long-term care users. Even where family or friends are available to care for someone with dementia, people may need additional support from formal care services. People who live at home may still need occasional help with basic activities of daily living, while those in residential care rely even more on professional support. While most countries have basic training programmes for professional health and social care staff, often these do not adequately prepare them for the challenges of caring well for someone with dementia. For example, public training on dementia is not available for caregivers in Greece. While non-governmental organisations, including Alzheimer Hellas, have offered training programmes to care professionals, these programmes are not official and do not provide accreditation.

Dementia-specific approaches that take a person-centred approach to caring are important to ensure that people with dementia receive good care. The Dementia ABC educational programme developed in Norway represents an example of how well-designed training programmes can be effectively integrated into existing health and social services to deliver high-quality care and improve job satisfaction. Developed by the Norwegian National Advisory Unit on Ageing and Health, the Dementia ABC programme is a two-year, interdisciplinary training programme open to professional staff working with people with dementia, across disciplines and levels of seniority. To promote engagement with the Dementia ABC programme, the Norwegian government, through the Norwegian national dementia plan, has engaged in a cost-sharing scheme with local municipalities. The programme is not targeted at a specific group of professionals, but is designed to be relevant for all who may engage with people with dementia in their work lives. Staff members who completed the educational programme were found to have increased their practice of person-centred care and exhibited improvements in job satisfaction.

Professional incentives can help with training uptake. Dementia-specific training programmes that teach care staff to respond effectively and empathetically can help improve well-being for the recipient of care. It can also improve the caregiver's experience. Some countries have incorporated dementia training into basic care, or developed training programmes that deliver additional expertise. For example, formal care workers are required to take additional dementia training to reach higher levels of qualification through the National Certificate in Health, Disability and Support in New Zealand. In some cases, dementia training is required to serve in certain care positions, such as dementia-aware home care workers in Belgium. Additional professional recognition and responsibility can help workers feel more engaged with and respected for the work they do.

Financial incentives can also encourage care workers to undertake additional training. In Norway, for example, home health aides and professional care staff who complete a vocational training course on dementia are eligible for higher salaries, while in New Zealand, the government has established minimum wage bands for care workers based on training and experience which are higher than the federal minimum wage. However, these examples remain the exception rather than the rule, and in most countries care staff is not professionally or financially rewarded for developing additional expertise in dementia care.

1.5.3. Inadequate hospital care for people with dementia can lead to worse outcomes for people with dementia

Many people with dementia will spend at least some time in an acute hospital, and it is important that hospitals are able to care for them in a way that minimises the stress of a hospital setting. But in most countries, it is far from clear that hospitals can accurately identify all or even most people with dementia who seek care. In a pilot analysis of hospital-based indicators collected by the OECD, many people who had previously received a dementia diagnosis did not have dementia recorded when they entered the hospital. This can affect not only the accuracy of hospital data, but also the quality of care the patient receives. Moreover, reducing hospital admissions is a worthy policy goal, but difficult to implement and evaluate when coding challenges remain so acute. A low admissions rate may indicate that a health system is indeed keeping people out of hospital, or it may conversely reflect a health system where diagnosis rates are poor, and many people do not receive the regular care they need.

Hospital coding standards that promote recording a dementia diagnosis should be improved. Coding standards that instruct health professionals on how to code diagnoses can impact how often diseases are recorded in hospital records. Many people with dementia may visit the hospital for a reason other than their dementia diagnosis. Where coding standards compel only conditions that need treatment during the current stay in hospital to be recorded, for example, dementia may not be recorded. This can happen even where a person has previously been diagnosed with dementia. Coding standards can significantly influence how specific diagnoses are recorded: in Australia, for example, the number of hospital admissions where dementia was recorded fell substantially following a change in coding standards in 2008. Even where dementia is not the primary reason for admission to hospital (as it rarely is), the condition can strongly impact the stay and can contribute to a worsening of health outcomes. For this reason, people with dementia would likely benefit from always having their diagnosis included in the hospital record, regardless of whether it is a reason for admission, or requires treatment at the time of admission.

Dementia is a progressive disease, and even when someone receives high-quality, person-centred care, there may still come a time when they need to seek acute care. A visit to the hospital can be a particularly distressing experience for someone with dementia, to the extent that many people leave the hospital doing less well than when they arrived (Sampson et al., 2009; Morrison and Siu, 2000; Nightingale et al., 2001). People with dementia may feel confused about where they are, and the sterile hospital setting and unfamiliar people can contribute to a heightened level of stress and agitation. People with dementia stay in hospital far longer than the overall average length of stay. Across the OECD, people with a diagnosis of dementia recorded in their hospital record stayed in hospital an average of 36 days, compared with just eight days for people who were not recorded to have dementia (OECD, 2017b). While people with dementia will sometimes need hospital care, the amount of time they stay in hospital should be reduced to the greatest extent possible. With adequate support, much of the care provided in hospitals can be provided at home. In the Netherlands, for example, a 'hospital at home' model of care admits people with dementia for only immediate treatment (such as surgery), while follow-up care is provided at home under the supervision of specialist nurses. Hospitals and health systems need to have strong connections with community-based and long-term care for such programmes to work well.

A major challenge of improving hospital care for people with dementia is that hospital staff may not recognise that a patient has dementia in the first place, as people are admitted to hospitals for other reasons than dementia – for example for a fracture following a fall. Even where someone has previously been diagnosed, a patient's medical history is often not fully communicated to the hospital. Where hospital staff is not aware of a dementia diagnosis, they may not be able to treat the patient using the best possible approach. Training programmes to teach hospital staff, and particularly those working in emergency departments, to recognise possible signs of dementia could help improve hospital care for people who were previously undiagnosed, or whose diagnosis was not conveyed to the hospital because patient records were not linked. Moreover, dementia is rarely the main cause of a hospital admission: in 2016, 98% of hospital admissions where dementia was coded had dementia coded as a secondary diagnosis in Israel, while 89% of admissions with a coding of dementia had dementia recoded as a secondary diagnosis in Sweden. This makes it even more important that a diagnosis of dementia is made before coming to hospital, and that this diagnosis is shared once admitted.

Inpatient mental health teams can help to manage behavioural challenges. The stress of a visit to the hospital for people with dementia can aggravate difficult behaviours or lead to delirium. Some countries have taken steps to moderate these harmful effects through specialised in-hospital dementia liaisons. Response teams to manage challenging behaviours are available in hospitals in Australia, while specialist mental health liaison teams provide support and advice to hospital staff on how to manage difficult behaviours in the United Kingdom and Slovenia. Upskilling all hospital staff to effectively manage BPSD may not be feasible, given the range of conditions staff encounter on a regular basis. In many cases, creating a small number of specialist positions to support the broader staff may be a more realistic approach.

1.5.4. People with dementia have insufficient access to end of life planning and care

The gradual decline and loss of function that define the disease's trajectory can make identifying the end of life stage of dementia particularly difficult. Without an ability to communicate their needs, people with dementia often reach the end stage of their life without access to the pain medication and palliative treatments that are more readily accessible to people with other diseases. In at least nine OECD countries, palliative care is unavailable or extremely difficult to access for people with dementia, even though it is more broadly available. Data on the availability of palliative care, particularly for people with dementia, is relatively poor. In Switzerland, a prospective study in the Swiss canton of Zurich is evaluating the end of life process for people with dementia, with a view to improving end of life care (Eicher et al., 2016).

Guidelines for palliative care should include dementia. Care staff may not be familiar with identifying the signs of end of life among people with dementia, or be unclear how palliative care should be administered when a patient is unable to communicate their preferences or needs. To date, no OECD country has developed a national framework for administering palliative care to people with dementia, though a number of countries, including the United Kingdom (England), Norway, and Switzerland, have identified people with dementia as a target group who need increased access.

By the end of their lives, people with dementia have often lost the ability to communicate with those around them, and are unable to understand the decisions that are made about them. This means that at the end of life, decisions may be taken about individuals' care that do not reflect what they would have wanted had they been able to express their preferences. Unable to express themselves, people with dementia may suffer from avoidable pain or discomfort. Advance care planning tools allow people with dementia to communicate their preferences in guidance or legally-binding directives before memory loss has taken hold.

Uptake of advanced care planning tools among people with dementia remains very low. Even where advance care planning is explicitly part of dementia care guidelines, health professionals may find it difficult to bring up the topic of end of life so quickly after a diagnosis. People with dementia and their families also find it difficult to discuss the end of life.

1.6. Conclusion

Most health and social care systems in OECD countries have focused attention on improving the quality of care for people with dementia, including by developing national policies and strategies to address dementia. Yet gaps in access to and the quality of services remain. More than half of people living with dementia remain undiagnosed, and fewer than 40% of countries can estimate rates of diagnosis nationally.

Despite the growing attention on the impact of dementia in OECD countries, data for dementia remains very poor, and little measurement of outcomes likely hampers efforts to improve the quality of care. Some of these weaknesses are related to broader data system challenges that cannot be addressed for dementia alone. Nevertheless, countries should take steps to improve the quality of dementia coding across the health system. The development of dementia registries can be considered to improve measurement where data systems are not adequately linked.

Given the importance of a diagnosis in facilitating access to services for dementia, this report recommends that countries continue their efforts to improve access to timely diagnosis for people with dementia. Primary care plays a growing role in diagnosing and caring for people with dementia, and primary care physicians require adequate training and support to ensure they perform these tasks well. Yet physicians average just twelve hours of dementia training during medical school, and no country has mandated dementia training as part of continuing medical education. As a consequence, primary care doctors often misdiagnose dementia, correctly identifying only around 50-75% of dementia cases.

More attention must also be paid to strengthening post-diagnostic services. Services are often dispersed across health and social care, as well as public, non-profit and private sectors. At least six countries – Australia, Denmark, Estonia, France, the Netherlands, and Norway – have developed specialised care pathways for people with early or complex dementia. Care co-ordination pathways and case management services are important to helping people with dementia – particularly those living at home – connect with the services available to them.

As people live at home longer, communities need to be better equipped to meet the needs of people living with dementia. Post-diagnostic care pathways can help connect people with dementia and their families with available services. But communities themselves must also adapt: community-friendly initiatives that train local populations and businesses to respond more effectively to people with dementia can help to reduce stigma around dementia while making the environment safer and more welcoming. Aging at home also means that informal carers will play an important role in supporting people with dementia. Informal carers should receive the support they need, and governments should assess whether existing services for carers are also adequate for carers of people with dementia, who may have unique needs.

Even where strong community-based support is offered, people with dementia will still sometimes need support from long-term care services and hospitals, particularly as dementia progresses. High rates of antipsychotic prescribing – averaging nearly 5% of people over 65 – suggests that the quality of care for people with behavioural and psychological symptoms of dementia should be further improved. New models of long-term care offer promising alternatives to traditional care facilities, and can be considered as the evidence for them is further developed. Lastly, structural barriers, including reimbursement, can sometimes hinder access to end of life palliative care services for people with dementia. Access to palliative care at the end of life should be strengthened, with special attention given to the needs of people with dementia.

References

Alzheimer's Disease International (2015), "World Alzheimer Report 2015: The Global Impact of Dementia – An Analysis of Prevalence, Incidence, Cost and Trends", Alzheimer's Disease International, London.

Björk, S. et al. (2016), "Exploring the prevalence and variance of cognitive impairment, pain, neuropsychiatric symptoms and ADL dependency among persons living in nursing homes; a cross-sectional study", *BMC Geriatrics*, Vol. 16, No. 1. https://dx.doi.org/10.1186%2Fs12877-016-0328-9.

Cannuscio, C. et al. (2002), "Reverberations of Family Illness: A Longitudinal Assessment of Informal Caregiving and Mental Health Status in the Nurses' Health Study", *American Journal of Public Health*, Vol. 92, No. 8, pp. 1305–1311. https://doi.org/10.2105/AJPH.92.8.1305.

Cowl, A.L. and J.E. Gaugler (2014), "Efficacy of creative arts therapy in treatment of Alzheimer's disease and dementia: a systematic literature review", *Activities, Adaptation & Aging*, Vol. 38, No. 4, pp. 281-330.

D'Onofrio, G. et al. (2014), "Caregiver burden characterization in patients with Alzheimer's disease or vascular dementia", *International Journal of Geriatric Psychiatry*, Vol. 30, pp. 891-899. https://doi.org/10.1002/gps.4232.

Eicher, S. et al. (2016), "The last phase of life with dementia in Swiss nursing homes: the study protocol of the longitudinal and prospective ZULIDAD study", *BMC Palliative Care*, Vol. 15, No. 1. https://doi.org/10.1186/s12904-016-0151-2.

Gallagher, D. et al. (2011), "Determinants of the desire to institutionalize in Alzheimer's caregivers", *American Journal of Alzheimer's Disease & Other Dementias*, Vol. 26, No. 3, pp. 205-211.

Gaugler, J. E. et al. (2009), "Predictors of Nursing Home Admission for Persons with Dementia", *Medical Care*, Vol. 47, No. 2, pp. 191–198.

Gomes, M. et al. (2017), "Cost-effectiveness of Memory Assessment Services for the diagnosis and early support of patients with dementia in England", *Journal of Health Services Research & Policy*, Vol. 22, No. 4, pp. 226–235. https://doi.org/10.1177/1355819617714816.

Kivipelto, M. et al. (2013), "The Finnish Geriatric Intervention Study to Prevent Cognitive Impairment and Disability (FINGER): study design and progress", *Alzheimer's & Dementia*, Vol. 9, No. 6, pp. 657-665.

Kivipelto, M., Mangialasche, F. and T. Ngandu (2018), "World Wide Fingers will advance dementia prevention", *The Lancet Neurology*, Vol. 17, No. 1, p. 27.

Knapp, M. et al. (2006), "Cognitive stimulation therapy for people with dementia: cost-effectiveness analysis", *British Journal of Psychiatry*, Vol. 188, pp. 574-580.

Knapp, M., Iemmi, V. and R. Romeo (2013), « Dementia care costs and outcomes : a systematic review", *International Journal of Geriatric Psychiatry*, Vol. 28, No. 6, pp. 551-561.

Kuzuya, M. et al. (2006), "Falls of the elderly are associated with burden of caregivers in the community", *International Journal of Geriatric Psychiatry*, Vol. 21, No. 8, pp. 740–745. https://doi.org/10.1002/gps.1554.

Langa, K.M. et al. (2017), "A comparison of the prevalence of dementia in the United States in 2000 and 2012", *JAMA Internal Medicine*, Vol. 177, No. 1, pp. 51-58.

Lesner, A.I. et al. (eds.) (2017), *Preventing cognitive decline and dementia: A way forward*, National Academies of Sciences, Engineering, and Medicine, The National Academies Press, Washington, D.C.

Livingston, G. et al. (2017), "Dementia prevention, intervention, and care", *The Lancet*, Vol. 390, No. 10113, pp. 1–62. https://doi.org/10.1016/S0140-6736(17)31363-6.

Matthews, F.E. et al. (2013), "A two-decade comparison of prevalence of dementia in individuals aged 65 years and older from three geographical areas of England: results of the Cognitive Function and Ageing Study I and II", *The Lancet*, Vol. 382, No. 9902, pp. 1405-1412.

Meeuwsen, E. J. et al. (2012), "Effectiveness of dementia follow-up care by memory clinics or general practitioners: randomised controlled trial", *BMJ*, Vol. 344, pp. e3086. https://doi.org/10.1136/bmj.e3086.

Mitchell, A. J., Meader, N. and M. Pentzek (2011), "Clinical recognition of dementia and cognitive impairment in primary care: a meta-analysis of physician accuracy", *Acta Psychiatrica Scandinavica*, Vol. 124, No. 3, pp. 165–183. https://doi.org/10.1111/j.1600-0447.2011.01730.x

Mittelman, M. S. et al. (2006), "Improving caregiver well-being delays nursing home placement of patients with Alzheimer disease", *Neurology*, Vol. 67, No. 9, pp. 1592–1599. https://doi.org/10.1212/01.wnl.0000242727.81172.91.

Morrison, R.S. and A.L. Siu (2000), "Survival in end-stage dementia following acute illness", *Journal of the American Medical Association*, Vol. 284, No. 1, pp. 47-52.

Ngandu, T. et al. (2015), "A 2 year multidomain intervention of diet, exercise, cognitive training, and vascular risk monitoring versus control to prevent cognitive decline in at-risk elderly people (FINGER): a randomised controlled trial", *The Lancet*, Vol. 385, No. 9984, pp. 2255-2263.

Nichols, L.O. et al. (2011), "Translation of a Dementia Caregiver Support Program in a Health Care System—REACH VA", *Archives of Internal Medicine*, Vol. 171, No. 4, pp. 353–359.

Nichols, L.O. et al. (2017), "Impact of the REACH II and REACH VA Dementia Caregiver Interventions on Healthcare Costs", *Journal of the American Geriatric Society*, Vol. 65, No. 5, pp. 931-936.

Nightingale, S. et al. (2001), "Psychiatric illness and mortality after hip fracture", *The Lancet*, Vol. 357, No. 9264, pp. 1264–1265. https://doi.org/10.1016/S0140-6736(00)04421-4.

OECD (2015a), *Addressing Dementia: The OECD Response*, OECD Health Policy Studies, OECD Publishing, Paris, http://dx.doi.org/10.1787/9789264231726-en.

OECD (2015b), *Health Data Governance: Privacy, Monitoring and Research*, OECD Health Policy Studies, OECD Publishing, Paris, http://dx.doi.org/10.1787/9789264244566-en.

OECD (2017a), *Health at a Glance 2017: OECD Indicators*, OECD Publishing, Paris, http://dx.doi.org/10.1787/health_glance-2017-en.

OECD (2017b), *OECD Health Statistics* (database), http://stats.oecd.org/index.aspx?DataSetCode=HEALTH_STAT.

Onder, G. et al. (2012), " Assessment of nursing home residents in Europe: the Services and Health for Elderly in Long TERm care (SHELTER) study", *BMC Health Services Research*, Vol. 12, No. 5. https://doi.org/10.1186/1472-6963-12-5.

Ory, M. G. et al. (1999), "Prevalence and Impact of Caregiving: A Detailed Comparison Between Dementia and Nondementia Caregivers", *The Gerontologist*, Vol. 39, No. 2, pp. 177–185.

Pinquart, M. and S Sörensen (2003), "Differences between caregivers and noncaregivers in psychological health and physical health: A meta-analysis.", *Psychology and Aging*, Vol. 18, No. 2, pp. 250–267. https://doi.org/10.1037/0882-7974.18.2.250.

Public Health Agency of Canada (2017), "Dementia in Canada, including Alzheimer's disease: Highlights from the Canadian Chronic Disease Surveillance System", available from https://www.canada.ca/content/dam/phac-aspc/documents/services/publications/diseases-conditions/dementia-highlights-canadian-chronic-disease-surveillance/dementia-highlights-canadian-chronic-disease-surveillance.pdf.

Russel, P. et al. (2013), "Improving the identification of people with dementia in primary care: evaluation of the impact of primary care dementia coding guidance on identified prevalence", *BMJ Open*, Vol. 3, No. e004023, https://doi.org/10.1136/bmjopen-2013-004023.

Sampson, E. L. et al. (2009), "Dementia in the acute hospital: prospective cohort study of prevalence and mortality", *The British Journal of Psychiatry*, Vol. 195, No. 1, pp. 61–66. https://doi.org/10.1192/bjp.bp.108.055335.

Sink, K.M. et al. (2006), "Caregiver characteristics are associated with neuropsychiatric symptoms of dementia", *Journal of the American Geriatrics Society*, Vol. 45, No. 5, pp. 796-803.

Spector, A. et al. (2003), "Efficacy of an evidence-based cognitive stimulation therapy programme for people with dementia: randomised controlled trial", *British Journal of Psychiatry,* Vol. 183, p. 248-254.

Spillman, B.C. and S.K. Long (2009), "Does High Caregiver Stress Predict Nursing Home Entry?", *Inquiry*, Vol. 46, pp. 140–161.

Spitznagel, M. B. et al. (2006), "Psychosocial Predictors of Dementia Caregiver Desire to Institutionalize: Caregiver, Care Recipient, and Family Relationship Factors", *Journal of Geriatric Psychiatry and Neurology*, Vol. 19, No. 1, pp. 16–20. https://doi.org/10.1177/0891988705284713.

Stansfeld, S. et al. (2014), "Stressors and common mental disorder in informal carers – An analysis of the English Adult Psychiatric Morbidity Survey 2007", *Social Science & Medicine*, Vol. 120, pp. 190-198.

Thomas, G.P.A. et al. (2015), "Informal carers' health-related quality of life and patient experience in primary care: evidence from 195,364 carers in England responding to a national survey", *BMC Family Practice*, Vol. 16, No. 62. https://doi.org/10.1186/s12875-015-0277-y.

Vaingankar, J.A. et al. (2016), "Care participation and burden among informal caregivers of older adults with care needs and associations with dementia", *International Psychogeriatrics*, Vol. 28, No. 2, pp. 221-231.

Vaughon, W. et al. (2018), "Association between falls and caregiving tasks among informal caregivers: Canadian Community Health Survey Data", *Canadian Journal on Aging*, Vol. 37, No. 1, pp. 70-75, https://doi.org/10.1017/S0714980817000496.

Waldorff, F.B. and S. Moller (2001), "Diagnostic evaluation of dementia in general practice in Denmark. A national survey", *Scandinavian Journal of Primary Health Care*, Vol. 19, No. 2, pp. 117–121. https://doi.org/10.1080/028134301750235367.

Waldorff, F.B. et al. (2003), "Implementation of a clinical dementia guideline", *Scandinavian Journal of Primary Health Care*, Vol. 21, No. 3, pp. 142-147. https://doi.org/10.1080/02813430310005136.

Wittenberg, R. et al. (2017), "Why no reliable estimate can be produced for the rate of return on investment in primary prevention of dementia", Public Health England, London, UK.

Yaffe, K. et al. (2002), "Patient and Caregiver Characteristics and Nursing Home Placement in Patients With Dementia", *The Journal of the American Medical Association*, Vol. 287, No. 16, pp. 2090–2098. https://doi.org/10.1001/jama.287.16.2090.

Chapter 2. Identifying people with dementia

This chapter reviews what countries are currently doing to better identify people living with dementia. Many people with dementia go too long without receiving a diagnosis, and when they are diagnosed, the information they receive – about the disease, and about the services available to help them – is often inadequate. In many cases, primary care has assumed an increasingly important role in diagnosis and care for dementia. Specialist services remain an important part of the diagnostic pathway in many countries, with memory clinics increasingly common in many OECD countries. Access to timely diagnosis remains poor, but better training and well-designed incentives for primary care physicians, improved standardisation of specialised services, and strengthened data linkages between health settings, can help ensure more people receive a diagnosis when they need it.

The statistical data for Israel are supplied by and under the responsibility of the relevant Israeli authorities. The use of such data by the OECD is without prejudice to the status of the Golan Heights, East Jerusalem and Israeli settlements in the West Bank under the terms of international law.

2.1. Access to timely diagnosis remains poor

Although there is no cure or disease modifying treatment for dementia, the outcomes that people with dementia and their families experience can be significantly improved by the right health and social care services. A diagnosis allows health professionals to direct people living with dementia and their families towards the services that will be most beneficial to them. Those with early dementia may be offered medications that improve symptoms, even if only temporarily. Psychosocial interventions such as cognitive stimulation therapy can help to improve cognition. Families and carers can be trained to provide better care for people with dementia and manage the impact of caring on themselves more effectively.

Developing and being diagnosed with dementia can be distressing for people with dementia and their families, so it is important that diagnoses are accurately detected and effectively communicated. But diagnosing dementia can be difficult in part because symptoms are hard to differentiate from other conditions such as depression (Robinson et al., 2015), and it is not always done well.

A *formal diagnosis* of dementia (see Box 2.1) is also required for access to certain services in some countries. Anti-dementia drugs such as anti-cholinesterase inhibitors almost always require a formal diagnosis of dementia prior to prescription. In many countries, a formal diagnosis means that people living with the disease can be reimbursed fully or partially for a range of social and clinical support services, including medications and home care.

Despite these benefits, diagnosis rates remain low. Many countries reported that half or more of all people with dementia are thought to be undiagnosed, leaving thousands of people without access to the health and social care services that could improve their lives. Improving these rates is crucial to the wellbeing of people with dementia and their families.

Box 2.1. What is a dementia diagnosis?

A "diagnosis" can mean different things in different countries and in different settings. At the simplest level, a diagnosis of dementia means someone is told by a health professional that, in their opinion, they have dementia. In this report, we refer to this type of interaction as an indicative diagnosis.

Where a diagnosis of dementia gives someone access to certain health and social care services, or additional reimbursement, this may require certain specific tests to be carried out, specialists to be consulted, or for the diagnosis to be made in a specified setting. In this report, we refer to a diagnosis that meets the criteria for accessing all relevant support in a certain country as a formal diagnosis. In some countries, there are no specified criteria for accessing support, so indicative and formal diagnoses would be the same.

2.1.1. Primary care doctors are central to diagnosis, but do not always have the skills and resources required to succeed in this role

Primary care is a central part of the dementia diagnostic process in most countries

Primary care doctors are the first point of contact for people with dementia in most countries. In nearly all OECD countries, people who are concerned that they might have dementia go first to their primary care doctor. Of 29 OECD countries reporting, 26 reported that primary care doctors are always or sometimes the first point of contact for dementia (see Table 2.1). The role of primary care in dementia detection is often formalised or highlighted in national dementia plans and strategies, including those of Australia, Chile, Denmark, Ireland, and Mexico, and is often linked with goals to promote timelier diagnosis.

In a small number of countries, people who think they might have dementia can bypass primary care and go directly to specialists. In Estonia, for example, primary care practitioners serve as only partial gatekeepers: while referrals are needed for consultations with neurologists, psychiatrists – who also diagnose dementia – can be consulted directly. Primary care practitioners similarly play only a small role in dementia diagnosis in Greece, with most patients bypassing the primary care system in favour of going directly to a neurologist or other specialist. In Germany, people can also directly access a specialist when symptoms of dementia are present. The Japanese health system does not register general practitioners in a separate category from specialists; insured patients are allowed to go directly to any physician (Nakanishi and Nakashima, 2014; OECD, 2015a).

In nearly all countries, primary care physicians perform at least a basic cognitive assessment and provide people with an indicative diagnosis. In the United Kingdom, for example, people with memory complaints will most commonly go first to their primary care physician. After conducting a simple memory test and basic blood tests to exclude other possible causes of cognitive problems, the general practitioner will in most cases refer the patient on to specialist care, such as a memory clinic or memory assessment service.

The actual role of the primary care physician in dementia care can vary from cursory screening and referral to a more comprehensive examination and care management. In nine countries, primary care doctors also provide a formal diagnosis (Table 2.1). In Chile, for example, a shortage of specialists in geriatrics and neurology has led to primary care being the focal point for all diagnostic services (as well as ongoing dementia management). However, in most countries the initial tests conducted by primary care physicians serve to rule out alternative explanations and confirm suspected cases of cognitive impairment for onward referral. People with suspected dementia are then referred to specialist services for further tests before a formal diagnosis is made.

Primary care doctors use a range of standardised tools and tests to assess people with suspected dementia (Box 2.2). The most common is the Mini Mental State Examination (MMSE), with the clock test and the Montreal Cognitive Assessment (MOCA), a screening tool for mild cognitive impairment also frequently administered at the primary care level. In some countries (Belgium, Denmark, and Sweden) blood tests are carried out in primary care to rule out other conditions that may mimic symptoms of dementia-related cognitive impairment. While more advanced testing and neuroimaging is most frequently administered by specialists, primary care physicians in Sweden and Norway have recently begun conducting CT scans as part of their initial screening process.

Primary care doctors are not always able to provide effective diagnostic services

In some cases primary care doctors lack the skills and experience to provide effective diagnostic services. For example, a survey of general practitioners in Denmark suggested that less than half of primary care practitioners were able to perform a good assessment of dementia (Waldorff and Moller, 2001). Other studies have found that primary care doctors correctly identify only around 75% of dementia cases, and often fail to record the diagnoses that they do make. The performance of primary care is worse with more complex cases, such as early-stage cognitive impairment (Mitchell et al., 2011).

Primary care doctors may also be reluctant to take on the central role that OECD health systems expect them to play in dementia diagnosis, because of a lack of confidence or a lack of capacity. An evaluation of diagnosis in primary care in the United Kingdom identified lack of confidence as a significant obstacle to diagnosing dementia in primary care (Dodd et al., 2014); while in Slovenia, a shortage of general practitioners has led to high patient loads and a reluctance to take on additional cases of dementia. There is also evidence that where clinicians feel little can be done to help people living with dementia, such as if they are unaware of existing treatments or local resources and services for people with dementia and their carers, they may be more reluctant to diagnose or communicate a diagnosis in the first place (Bradford et al., 2009).

Table 2.1. Dementia diagnosis roles carried out by primary care physicians

	First point of contact	Indicative diagnosis	Formal diagnosis	Initiating medications
Australia	X	X	X	X
Austria	X	X		
Belgium	X	X		
Canada (British Columbia)	X	X	X	X
Chile	X	X	X	X
Czech Republic	X	X		
Denmark	X	X	X	
Estonia	X			
Finland	X	X		
France	X	X		
Germany	X	X		
Greece		X		
Hungary	X			
Ireland	X	X		
Israel	X	X		
Luxembourg	X	X		
Mexico	X	X		
Netherlands	X	X	X	X
New Zealand	X	X	X	X
Norway	X	X	X	X
Portugal	X	X		
Slovak Republic	X	X		
Slovenia	X	X		
Sweden	X	X	X	X
Switzerland	X	X	X	X
Turkey				
United Kingdom (England)	X	X	In some cases (rare)	
United States	X	X		

Source: OECD Dementia Survey and Interviews 2016-2017.

Box 2.2. Detecting dementia in primary care

As the role of general practitioners in assessment and diagnosis of dementia has grown, a range of cognitive assessment tools have been developed to assist physicians in determining whether their patients have become cognitively impaired. Some assessment tools, such as the general practitioner assessment of cognition, have been developed specifically to be used in primary care settings. The most widely used cognitive impairment screening tools share a number of common characteristics: they are short (intended to be used within a regular doctor's visit), easy to administer, and easy to score. The design of different screening tools nevertheless introduces different biases into the assessment, including related to level of education, cultural background, and how symptoms of dementia or cognitive impairment manifest in different people.

Mini mental state exam (MMSE)

The MMSE is a 30-point, 11-question assessment that tests cognitive function in the areas of orientation, registration, attention and calculation, recall, language, and visual construction. Originally proposed in 1975, it is the most frequently used cognitive assessment tool for dementia. While easy to administer, it is judged to be less effective for detecting mild cognitive impairment, while its structure – notably its use of verbal responses and written questions – may contribute to performance biases based on education level and language fluency. Unlike most cognitive assessment tools, the MMSE is copyrighted, somewhat limiting its use. Because of its copyright, the MMSE is somewhat less frequently recommended as an assessment tool in clinical guidelines.

General practitioner assessment of cognition

The general practitioner assessment of cognition was explicitly developed for use in primary care. It can be completed in less than five minutes and includes both a cognitive assessment of the patient and, in certain cases, a questionnaire for a family member or carer.

Montreal cognitive exam

The Montreal Cognitive Exam (MoCA) is a 10-minute, 30-point exam designed to screen for cognitive impairment. Scores from MoCA and the MMSE have found to be similar, particularly for people with dementia, though a number of studies indicate that MoCA may be more sensitive in detecting cases of earlier (mild) cognitive impairment (Nasreddine et al., 2005, Zadikoff et al., 2008, Dong et al., 2010, Trzepacz et al., 2015).

Memory impairment screen

The memory impairment screen is a four-minute delayed and cued recall test to evaluate memory impairment. Its short length and straightforward scoring make it easy to administer and evaluate. It is considered to be as sensitive as the MMSE in detecting cognitive impairment, though it does not assess cognitive impairment in the domains of visuospacial ability or executive function.

Mini cognitive assessment instrument

The mini-cognitive assessment ("mini-cog") is a three-minute, three-part test that incorporates recall and delayed recall exercises with a clock test drawing. Its simplicity and brevity may be advantageous compared with longer assessment tools, such as the MMSE, given the short appointment times primary care practitioners often have with their patients. The mini-cog has been found to be as sensitive as the MMSE and other assessment tools in detecting cognitive impairment (Borson et al., 2003).

2.1.2. Guidelines are important to improving diagnosis in primary care

Many countries have developed clinical guidelines to improve dementia diagnosis in primary care

A number of countries have taken steps to promote high quality dementia diagnosis and care through the development of guidelines. Guidelines frequently include recommended assessment tools for diagnosis, principles of communation and care, and in some cases recommended pathways for care following referral or diagnosis. At least 16 OECD countries have guidelines for dementia diagnosis and care (see Table 2.2).

In some cases, guidelines have been developed specifically for, or tailored to, the primary care setting, as in NHS England's *Dementia diagnosis and management: a brief pragmatic resource for general practitioners*. Similar primary care-specific guidelines are being developed in Belgium (by the University of Leuven) and Switzerland (by the Association of Swiss Memory Clinics).

Table 2.2. Countries with clinical guidelines for dementia management

	Clinical guidelines	Clinical guidelines apply to or directed at primary care
Australia	Yes	Yes
Belgium	No	In development
Canada (British Columbia only)	Yes	Yes
Chile	Yes	Yes
Czech Republic	No official, nationally disseminated guidelines	No
Denmark	Yes	Yes
Estonia	Yes	No
Finland	Yes	Yes
France	Yes	Yes
Germany	Yes	Yes
Greece	No	No
Hungary	No	No
Ireland	No	No
Israel	No	No
Luxembourg	No	No
Mexico	Yes	Yes
Netherlands	Yes	Yes
New Zealand	Yes	Yes
Norway	Yes	Yes
Portugal	No	No
Slovak Republic	Yes	
Slovenia	No	No
Sweden	Yes	Yes
Switzerland	Yes	Under development
Turkey	No	No
United Kingdom (England)	Yes	Yes
United States	Yes (not federal)	Yes

Publicising guidelines and providing better training can help primary care doctors to comply with best practice

While guidelines can serve as a useful information resource for physicians, they are non-binding and may not always be followed. This may simply be because primary care doctors are not aware that guidelines exist or do not know where to find them. In many countries, guidelines are not developed by one single clinical body but may be produced by medical associations, nongovernmental bodies, or other associations. In the United States, for example, the Gerontological Society of America convened a Workgroup on Cognitive Impairment Detection and Earlier Diagnosis and developed a toolkit to help primary care physicians detect cognitive impairment and diagnose dementia (Gerontological Society of America, 2017). Publicising the existence of guidelines to primary care doctors may therefore help to improve compliance. However, there is also evidence that where doctors feel that they lack the skills to apply the recommendations found in guidelines, they may disregard them (de Lepeleire et al., 2008). This suggests that, to be effective, guidelines must be supported by training.

2.1.3. Adequate training for primary care doctors is essential for improving diagnosis

Across the OECD, primary care physicians have access to at least some dementia training, either during medical school or as part of their continuing education. Dementia training during undergraduate or graduate medical school remains limited. In most countries, primary care physicians are required to maintain their skills through a minimum number of continuing education hours per year. Training in dementia management is offered as an option to fulfil these requirements in many of these countries, including in Australia, Austria, Belgium, Hungary, the Netherlands, New Zealand, Sweden, and the United States.

Dementia training tends to be limited during medical school, though continuing education on dementia is available in most countries

Dementia training during undergraduate or graduate medical school remains limited, with many countries reporting that medical students receive very little training – often just one or two days – during their studies. Across 10 European countries, medical students average just 12 hours of dementia training during their studies (Tsolaki et al., 2010). In almost all countries, additional training on dementia is offered as part of continuing education programmes. . While training for dementia care is often offered as one of a suite of continuing education programmes available to primary care physicians, and can satisfy minimum continuing certification requirements, the choice of training topics are usually left to the clinician. Enrolling in dementia courses often requires clinicians to spend extra hours in training, which can result in lost income or cut into free time. Courses – particularly when offered by nongovernmental organisations – may also rely on external financing, including support from employers or municipalities. Where such reimbursement is not forthcoming, participation may suffer.

However, few incentives and barriers to participation mean take-up can be low and participation relies largely on the personal or professional interests of the physicians. Though they can help to increase participation rates, incentives for participating in dementia training are offered in very few OECD countries. The few incentives that are promoted focus primarily on either financial reimbursement or special certification rewards. Primary care physicians in Denmark do not have any continuing education requirements to practice, though training programmes are widely available. A reimbursement scheme has been developed that allows primary care practitioners, as well as specialists in private practice, to be reimbursed for the income they lose while undergoing training.

Developing nationally-available, dedicated dementia training courses may be another way to expand the reach of dementia training programmes and increase quality of care. In 2016, Australia launched a national training program providing dementia training to primary care providers, acute care, and aged care providers across specialities and levels of experience. Courses cover a range of issues, including diagnosis and care, medications management, and managing behavioural and psychiatric symptoms of dementia (BPSD). The training courses, which comprise a suite of options ranging from online short courses to tertiary-level qualifications, are administered by a consortium that includes five Australian universities, as well as the nongovernmental organisation Dementia Australia. In Denmark, the Danish Dementia Research Centre, the Danish Medical Association, and other providers offer both in-person and online training to primary health physicians and other health professionals.

Working with the Swedish Dementia Centre, the Karolinska Institute launched a Master's in Dementia Care for Physicians in 2012, a web-based, part-time two-year program for physicians intended to improve dementia management for themselves and their clinics. The program requires all students to be funded by their employers. In Sweden, demand for the program from physicians has outstripped the willingness to pay by county councils, who are responsible for financing continuing education. The program has also accepted students from abroad, including from Japan and Germany.

Online training courses can reach more doctors more cheaply, but may not deliver the same outcomes

Online training programmes are increasingly used to increase access to information about dementia management that accommodates health professionals' geographic or time restraints. In Mexico, the government recently launched a massive open online course (MOOC) focusing on dementia management. It has so far reached 5 000 health professionals, including primary care physicians, since its launch. Some of New Zealand's continuing education training programmes are available later as online resources. The Danish Dementia Research Centre has identified e-learning as a key opportunity for training and knowledge dissemination (Tannebaek et al., 2014). More than 600 primary care practitioners – more than 15% of the country's primary care physicians – have participated in an ABC e-learning module launched by the Research Centre in November 2016. When appropriately designed, e-learning modules may also help to reduce quality discrepancies between programmes, by allowing a large number of participants to benefit from the same, carefully designed curriculum.

Offering internet-based training courses can expand the reach of dementia education to a broader population of physicians and health professionals, though the quality of online courses and their impact on physician practice may not be as strong as more traditional training approaches. While even short-term training programmes may help increase physician's confidence in their ability to care for people with dementia, there is some evidence to suggest that in-person training programmes and decision support interventions may be more effective than individual e-learning (Downs et al., 2006, Lathren et al., 2013).

Providing more intensive training to a small number of doctors may be a more realistic strategy to ensure access to expertise

Despite the increasing prevalence of dementia, not all primary care services will treat a high volume of cases Training all primary care physicians in dementia care management may not be the best use of limited resources if caseloads for many are low. And even where physicians see a large number of older patients – as is increasingly the case across OECD countries given rapid population aging – a policy that tries to increase the skill level of all doctors equally will only be able to cover basic dementia care training, and risks increasing skill level only marginally.

Investing resources to intensively upskill a limited number of primary care physicians may be a more effective approach. Physicians who express particular interest in dementia, or those who have a high caseload of older patients, could be targeted to receive additional training. In concert with more broadly available dementia training courses for primary care practitioners, a number of OECD countries have begun developing training programmes that aim to strengthen cooperation between primary care physicians and harness individual knowledge to improve dementia management across clinics. Together with an umbrella organisation of general practitioners, the University of Leuven in Belgium has begun developing a program that would identify and train specific primary care physicians to act as "reference" physicians for dementia for other practitioners handling fewer cases of dementia. In Mexico, a six-month training program targeting primary care professionals (including both physicians and nurses) takes place largely online. The program also includes an in-person training component with other participants, with the explicit purpose of developing a network of health professionals trained in dementia management.

2.1.4. Population screening for dementia is uncommon, but increasing

In an effort to promote early detection and increase diagnosis rates, countries have undertaken population screening programmes for a number of diseases, such as breast cancer and colon cancer. Population screening has proven to be a popular approach in OECD countries when detection rates for various diseases are suboptimal. Across the OECD, for example, more than three-fifths of women are screened for breast cancer (OECD, 2017). Unlike screening programmes for cancers, where the evidence relating to improved outcomes from early detection and treatment is more developed, the effectiveness of screening programmes for dementia is much less clear. Countries have largely refrained from or actively rejected implementing population screening programmes to detect dementia, despite persistently low diagnosis rates.

The effectiveness of screening programmes for dementia is unclear

Concerns about developing population screening programmes for dementia rest largely on the insufficient evidence of effect they have demonstrated, and the lack of cure for the disease. With no prospect for a cure, receiving a diagnosis before a person is ready to may lead to substantial emotional and psychological distress, with little additional benefit (Lecouteur et al., 2013, Turner, 2013, Mate et al., 2017). When people with dementia receive a diagnosis they are not expecting – which can particularly be the case for people with early and mild forms of the disease – the news can have a devastating effect.

Furthermore, there is no guarantee that people diagnosed through screening programmes will receive adequate follow-up care after diagnosis. Treatment options for dementia are extremely limited already, and there is some evidence suggesting that the follow-up action and care patients receive after a diagnosis through screening is low, particularly for younger patients and people with less than severe cognitive impairment (Boustani et al., 2005, Borson et al., 2007).

Screening programmes also run the risk of mistakenly identifying people without dementia as having the disease. General population screening programmes, even when restricted to older populations, have been found to have false-positive screening rates that may be as high as one in five among those initially screened positive for cognitive impairment. Because of the low prevalence of dementia in the general population, the positive predictive value of the screening assessments will also be lower in a general screening program than in more targeted settings (Boustani et al., 2005, Mate et al., 2017). The additional costs of screening, lack of preparedness of primary care physicians to undertake such screening programmes, and the additional time burden have further been identified as arguments against implementing broader screening programmes for dementia.

General population screening for dementia is uncommon, though some countries have recently introduced programmes

Most OECD countries have not implemented general population screening programmes for dementia. In a number of countries, including the United Kingdom and Australia, national clinical guidelines advise against the practice, while others, including the United States, have concluded that current evidence is insufficient to develop further recommendations (LeCouteur et al., 2013, U.S. Preventive Services Task Force, 2014, UK National Screening Committee, 2015, Guideline Adaptation Committee, 2016).

Nevertheless, four countries reported that they have developed cognitive screening programmes for older populations: Chile, Finland, South Korea, and the United States (Table 2.3). South Korea has implemented national population screening for dementia through the National Dementia Early Detection Program (NDEDP) since 2010. As part of its goal of strengthening its diagnostic system for dementia, Chile has similarly planned to integrate a clinical evaluation for dementia into its annual preventive health exam for older adults, the Examen de Medicina Preventiva del Adulto Mayor (EMPAM) (Chilean Ministry of Health, 2015). Three communities were selected to begin implementing the country's dementia plan in primary care in 2017.

Cognitive screening was recently introduced to Medicare recipients in the United States. Under the Patient Protection and Affordable Care Act (ACA), Medicare recipients are entitled to an annual Wellness Visit, which includes an assessment to detect "any cognitive impairment" (Hughes et al 2011, Borson et al., 2013). Some concerns have been raised over the possibility of an increase in false positives as a result of this program; to help reduce this risk, clinicians have proposed a short screening indicator to help general practitioners identify patients at high-risk of cognitive impairment (Barnes et al., 2014).

Other countries have considered developing screening programmes, or have plans to do so. In the Czech Republic, a two-year pilot project has seen general practitioners include basic dementia screening, including blood tests and a mini-cog examination, in biennial preventative exams available to all patients above the age of 60. The Ministry of Health is also in the process of developing a special project focused on expanding preventative screening programmes beyond cancer, and is considering dementia screening as one possible option. Beginning in, 2019, screening for dementia will also be rolled out in primary care in Turkey, as part of its efforts toward the earlier detection of dementia.

Table 2.3. Screening programmes for dementia

	National screening?
Australia	No
Austria	No
Belgium	No
Canada (British Columbia)	No
Chile	Yes
Czech Republic	Pilot
Denmark	No
Estonia	No
Finland	Memory screening for all over 75+
France	No
Greece	No
Hungary	No
Ireland	No
Israel	Screening at 75 in one HMO
Korea	Yes
Luxembourg	No
Mexico	No
Netherlands	No
New Zealand	No
Norway	No
Portugal	No
Slovak Republic	No
Slovenia	No
Sweden	No
Switzerland	No
Turkey	Starting in 2019
United Kingdom	No
United States	Cognitive screening through Medicare Wellness Visit

Source: OECD Dementia Survey and Interviews 2016-2017.

Future medical advancements could change the benefit-risk calculation behind population screening for dementia

The balance of harms and benefits of population screening may change in the coming years. More recently, the question of whether countries should develop general population screening programmes has been revived by advancements in the understanding of the onset of dementia. After a number of promising anti-dementia medications, including Eli Lilly's solanezumab and Merck's verubecestat, failed during late-stage clinical trials, researchers have increasingly focused on developing treatments for dementia that must be administered years before any symptoms emerge. A number of ongoing clinical trials are testing this theory by administering anti-dementia medications in pre-symptomatic populations. Initial results will likely be published in 2019 and 2020. Should these interventions work, governments will be faced with new questions over how to identify the populations that would best benefit from these new disease-modifying treatments.

2.2. Specialist services continue to play an important role in diagnosing dementia

Even with the increasing focus placed on primary care management for dementia, formal diagnosis continues to take place at the specialist level, and often in memory clinics, in nearly all countries. The reasons for referral to specialists can vary, but can include primary physicians being unwilling to make a formal diagnosis, the need for a differential diagnosis, or insurance requirements that dementia be formally diagnosed by a specialist before available support can be accessed.

Specialists are needed to identify dementia sub-types and may often be more experienced in caring for people with dementia, including identifying the best available treatment options and local services available to a person with dementia and their family. Neurologists, psychiatrists, and geriatricians, are often needed to diagnose specific sub-types of dementia, including Alzheimer's disease, dementia with Lewy Bodies, and vascular dementia. Receiving a differential (sub-type) dementia diagnosis is important to ensure the best treatment pathways can be adopted. Different dementia sub-types have been found to respond differently to existing dementia treatment options, including memantine and anti-cholinesterase inhibitors (Livingston et al., 2017).

2.2.1. The availability of specialists varies significantly across OECD countries

Following a visit with a primary care physician, people suspected of having dementia are regularly referred to a specialist – most frequently geriatricians, psychiatrists, and neurologists – for further testing and to confirm the diagnosis. However, the number of specialists ranges substantially across OECD countries, indicating access to specialist care is not always consistent. For psychiatrists and neurologists, physician density varies more than three-fold across the OECD, with just 17 per 100 000 in Portugal, compared with 57 per 100 000 in Switzerland (see Figure 2.1).

Figure 2.1. Specialist density per 100 000 population

2015 (or nearest year)

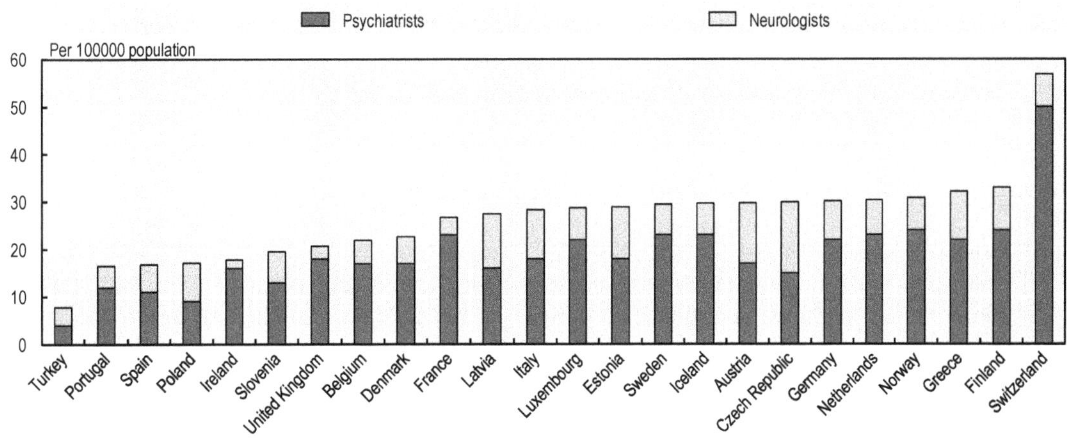

Source: OECD Health Statistics 2017, http://dx.doi.org/10.1787/health-data-en ; Eurostat Database 2018.

StatLink http://dx.doi.org/10.1787/888933735177

To facilitate diagnosis, many countries have set up specialist memory clinics to help with diagnosis and care. As attention to dementia management has grown in OECD countries, the role of the memory clinic has taken an increasingly prominent position in national plans or strategies, and in some cases formalised diagnostic pathways. While specialists can also operate independently, in the past decades the memory clinic structure has emerged as an important component of diagnosis or care for people with dementia. Of the 31 OECD countries interviewed for this report, only six countries – the Czech Republic, Estonia, Hungary, the Slovak Republic, Slovenia, and Turkey – reported having no memory clinics in their country. Between 1993 and 2000, the number of memory clinics in the United Kingdom more than doubled, from 20 to 58 (Lindesay et al., 2002). As of 2017, there are approximately 200 memory clinics in England. Similarly, of eight memory clinics identified in New Zealand in 2008, six had been established within the previous five years (Cheung and Strachan, 2008).

Box 2.3. What is a memory clinic?

Despite the rising profile of memory clinics in dementia care, what a memory clinic is has different interpretations in different settings. Originally memory clinics served as specialised clinical settings where health professionals – often neurologists, geriatricians, or psychiatrists – provided advanced diagnostic services.

In this report, we define *memory clinics* most broadly as any clinical setting where health professionals provide advanced diagnostic services and define themselves, or are defined externally (such as by insurance companies), as memory clinics. More specifically, we consider clinics that provide diagnostic services but no or only limited follow-up care to be *diagnostic memory clinics*. Memory clinics that are integrated into defined care pathways or otherwise engage in care management, education or training, and other components of dementia care are defined here as *comprehensive memory clinics*.

Few countries have developed clear guidelines or definitions around the staff profile, organisational structure, or location of memory clinics, or the services that they are expected to deliver. Consequently, most countries have a mix of diagnostic and comprehensive memory clinics. In some countries, the services provided by memory clinics may be case-dependent, or otherwise not clearly defined, in which case the broadest definition will be used.

Memory clinics play a major role in formal and differential diagnosis

Memory clinics operate as diagnostic centres for at least some cases of dementia in nearly all countries. A formal assessment at a memory clinic has become part of the recommended diagnostic pathway in some countries. Guidelines by the National Institute for Health and Care Excellence (NICE) in the United Kingdom identify memory assessment services as the "single point of referral for people with possible dementia" following a primary care assessment (NICE, 2006). Memory clinics are sometimes the only setting available for specialist consultation related to dementia. For example, Denmark has no geriatric specialists in private practice, while neurologists and psychiatrists in private practice almost never accept patients with dementia. While there are some neurologists and psychiatrists in private practice, they almost never take cases of dementia. As a result, people suspected of having dementia are nearly always referred to a memory clinic if follow-up specialist assessment or care is needed.

In some circumstances, memory clinics have been identified on the diagnostic pathway as important points of referral for more complex cases of dementia. Complex or rare cases of dementia can include dementia in younger persons, early stage dementia, people presenting with complex comorbidities, and people with minority language or cultural backgrounds. In Norway, people with suspected cases of dementia are recommended to be seen by their primary care physician and the municipal memory team. New guidelines further recommend that complex or unusual cases be referred to a memory clinic. In the Netherlands, where primary care is encouraged to participate in dementia care management to the greatest possible extent, both memory clinics and even more highly specialised university Alzheimer's centres are available for diagnostic support, care, treatment, and research for people with complex or difficult cases.

Some countries have developed specific services for people with early onset dementia. People with early onset dementia – which is characterized by the development of dementia before the age of 65 – often face a different or additional set of challenges to those experienced by older people with the condition. Among other considerations, they and their carers may still be working. In France, a special national reference centre dedicated to people with early onset dementia has been established to address their unique needs and ensure they have access to clinical services and adapted support throughout their lives.

The characteristics, concentration and distribution of memory clinics differs between countries

In most cases, memory clinics in OECD countries are multi-disciplinary and led by specialists. A review of memory clinics by Jolley, Benbow and Grizzel (2006) identified a number of common specialist settings for memory clinics, including psychiatry, neurology, and geriatrics, with most clinics based in geriatric psychiatry services (Cheung and Strachan, 2008; Lindesay et al., 2002). One or more of these specialties is found in most memory clinics in the OECD. In Austria, memory clinics are typically led by a neurologist or psychiatrist, who works alongside a psychologist and nurse in making diagnoses and sometimes offer further post-diagnostic support to people with dementia and their families. Greek memory clinics are similarly structured, with the majority led by neurologists working in concert with psychologists and nurses. Memory clinics in Israel are most commonly run by neurologists or geriatricians and often supported by a multidisciplinary team that can include neuropsychologists, psychiatrists, nurses and social workers. In England, memory clinics are normally led by old age psychiatrists, with support from medics, nurses, psychologists, and neuropsychologists. Unlike in most other health care systems, neurologists play a very small role in diagnosing and care for dementia in Norway, where specialists more often come from geriatrics or psychiatry. In the eight memory clinics in New Zealand identified in a review by Cheung and Strachan (2008), psychogeriatricians, geriatricians, psychologists, and occupational therapists were found to act as lead clinicians. No memory clinics were led by neurologists.

Specialists most likely to diagnose and care for people with dementia can differ geographically. In the north of Sweden, for example, geriatricians typically lead memory clinics, while in the south, psychiatrists are more common. There is similar regional variation in New Zealand. In most cases, whether a person with dementia sees a neurologist, geriatrician, or psychiatrist depends less on their symptoms and more on the staff profile of nearby memory clinics.

As many as 25 out of 31 OECD countries interviewed for this report have developed memory clinics. Data from countries with longitudinal information indicate that clinics have also expanded rapidly in recent years. The number of memory clinics doubled in the United Kingdom between 1993 and 2000 and quadrupled in New Zealand between 2003 and 2008. In France, 28 resource and research memory centres for complex and atypical cases and 500 to 600 memory consultation centres provide diagnostic services for people suspected of having dementia. The number of people aged 65 and over per memory clinic varies widely across countries, from more than 170 000 people 65 and over per memory clinic in Belgium to about 23 000 per memory clinic in France (Table 2.4). While the concentration of memory clinics within countries likely also differs, this national variation also indicates that different countries rely to different extents on memory clinics as a part of the clinical pathway for dementia.

Table 2.4. Population 65+ per memory clinic (thousands)

Australia	155
Belgium	171
Denmark	28
France	23
Ireland	33
Italy	27
Netherlands	30
New Zealand	113
OECD(10)	65
Sweden	32
Switzerland	42

Note: The organisation and definition of memory clinics differs between countries, and may not be directly comparable.
Source: 2017 OECD Dementia Care Policy Interviews (Belgium, New Zealand, Switzerland, Ireland, Sweden, the Netherlands, Denmark, and Italy). Data for Australia: Woodward and Woodward, 2009.

Few countries have developed guidelines and standards to help define the role of memory clinics

Almost no OECD countries have developed official definitions related to the operations of memory clinics. This has led to significant variation in the services offered by clinics both between and within countries. An important exception is France, which has developed guidelines outlining requirements for both its *Centres Mémoire de Ressource et de Recherche (CMRR)* and *Centres Mémoire (CM)*. In the absence of national or regional guidelines, the comprehensiveness of care offered in a memory clinic often depends on the interests and capacities of the managing physician and their connection to nearby services. In Switzerland, the Swiss Memory Clinics association has had quality standards for admission into the association since 2011. A similar network of memory clinics was recently set up in the Netherlands. The Dutch Memory Clinic Network was launched in 2016 to promote knowledge sharing and improve care across memory clinics. As part of its work, standards for memory clinics are in the process of being developed. In the United Kingdom, the Memory Services National Accreditation Programme accredits memory services that meet national guidelines, including the NICE Quality Standard for Dementia (Royal College of Psychiatrists 2018).

Box 2.4. Developing guidelines for memory clinics in Switzerland and Denmark

Guidelines for memory clinics developed in Switzerland and Denmark can be seen as "minimum standards" that ensure clinics provide quality services that reflect national or globally developed standards, particularly for diagnosis. Both guidelines cover the minimum caseload expected of clinics, as well as the professional composition of memory clinic teams.

Swiss Memory Clinics Association

In order to be considered for membership, memory clinics must demonstrate that they conduct at least 100 diagnostic evaluations for dementia every year. Evaluations must be comprehensive and multi-modal, and diagnosis must be established with interdisciplinary consultation. Four professional disciplines must be available through the memory clinic: geriatrics, geriatric psychiatry, neurology, and neuropsychology. In addition, memory clinics must comply with national and international recommendations and engage in public awareness and network-building with the community and other related services. 12 process-oriented quality standards have been developed to ensure that memory clinics meet standards of membership.

Danish Memory Clinic Guidelines

Recently published guidelines from the National Health Board of Denmark are directed at the changes to existing memory clinics the five administrative regions of the country are expected to make to qualify for additional financing for memory clinics under the National Plan. The guidelines recommend that each memory clinic serve a population of at least 300 000 people and conduct a minimum of 400, but preferably at least 500, diagnostic evaluations each year. Memory clinics should have neurologists, psychiatrists, geriatricians, neuropsychologists, and nurses on staff. Add more once guidelines are out. The guidelines are partially based on the experiences developing memory clinics in the capitol region of Denmark.

2.2.2. Services at memory clinics can vary widely, though many have begun to take on roles beyond diagnosis

In recent years, diagnostic memory clinics have expanded beyond their initial role as a location for detailed diagnostic assessment, and increasingly provide post-diagnostic support services and care for people with dementia throughout their lives. In addition to 'traditional' diagnostic memory clinics, new models of clinic-based care have begun to emerge in many OECD countries.

Box 2.5. What is post-diagnostic support?

After receiving a diagnosis of dementia, people living with dementia and their families and carers must adjust to what can be a crushing diagnosis. A range of resources – from health services, social services, and the nongovernmental sector –are often available to help them with daily living activities, emotional and social support, information and training, advanced care planning, and other needs. Yet in many cases, these available services are fragmented, and people with dementia may not receive adequate information about what these services are, their relevance, and how to access them. In the worst case, a person with dementia may be sent home with a diagnosis and no information related to what this means or what to do moving forward. To avoid this outcome, many countries have begun to pay attention to strengthening the co-ordination of care that occurs after a person has received a diagnosis. Post-diagnostic support refers to the kind of support – in terms of care, services, resources, and co-ordination – that a person with dementia receives in the aftermath of a diagnosis.

Some comprehensive memory clinics emphasise the role of other health professionals, including primary care physicians and nurses. Others do not identify as memory clinics but offer many of the same services, often with a greater emphasis on holistically caring for the person with dementia and their families. As interest in the role of memory clinics has increased, the services provided by some clinics have expanded beyond diagnosis, to increasingly include post-diagnostic treatment, case management, support for families of people with dementia, and education and training services for health professionals or the broader community. In England, for example, memory clinics work closely with the Alzheimer's Society. Dementia support workers and dementia care advisors may be present at the memory clinic, or are otherwise available to signpost people with dementia and their families to post-diagnostic support.

Comprehensive clinic models have moved away from diagnostic services to focus more broadly on dementia care

In the past years, memory clinics have increasingly moved away from a focus on diagnostics to also play an active role in dementia care management, through a model that can be conceptualised more broadly as *comprehensive memory clinics*. One such model has seen memory clinics expand to the primary care level. In Ontario, Canada, a shortage of geriatricians has created serious capacity constraints and high waiting times for specialist consultation. Across Canada, there were just 261 registered geriatricians in 2015, a rate of 0.7 per 100 000 population, compared with nearly 3 000 paediatricians (Canadian Medical Association, 2015, Canadian Medical Association, 2016). As one response, physicians developed a model of primary care-based dementia detection and management (Lee et al., 2014). Part-time memory clinics were established within existing family health teams (FHT), a collaborative model that consists of family physicians, nurses, and social workers delivering primary care in local communities. Memory clinics are led by family physicians who have received additional training in diagnosing and caring for dementia, with the explicit aim of reducing reliance on geriatrics and other specialty services in not only care, but also diagnosis (Lee et al., 2011). Geriatricians or geriatric psychiatrists provide additional consultative support to the family physicians as needed. In an evaluation of 16 family health teams operating memory clinics, a review by geriatricians of diagnoses made by primary care practitioners found high agreement with their evaluations and subsequent care management plans (Lee et al., 2014). Just 8.9% of patients were referred to a specialist, compared with referral rates of over 80% among regular primary care physicians (Lee et al., 2014).

A similar approach to primary care-led memory clinics has been taken in the England. Beginning in 2006, the Gnosall Primary Care Clinic in Staffordshire has run a monthly memory clinic in its primary care facilities with an aim to increase diagnosis rates and reduce waiting times between the identification of symptoms and diagnosis (Benbow et al., 2013). As in Ontario, the memory clinic operates part-time and is located within a broader primary care clinic. Unlike the Ontario model, where the primary care physicians lead diagnosis, the Gnosall Primary Care Memory Clinic incorporates a geriatric psychiatrist into the practice staff at the memory clinic. Following the identification of suspected cases of dementia by the general practitioner, consultant geriatric psychiatrists review health care records and see the patient and their family members during the memory clinic visit. By situating the memory clinic within the existing primary care practice, proponents of the model argue that the consultant specialists can more thoroughly review the patient's medical history before the consultation (Benbow et al., 2013). In addition, the familiar location of the memory clinic is seen as advantageous in facilitating a lower-stress environment in which to receive the diagnosis (Benbow et al., 2013). The Gnosall Primary Care Memory Clinic has further developed the role of an 'eldercare facilitator' to help coordinate between the staff of the memory clinic and external agencies and services (Greaves et al., 2015). A review of the Gnosall model found that, compared with similar practices in the region, the primary care-based memory clinic resulted in higher satisfaction among people with their dementia and their families, lower utilisation of other health care services, and substantial cost-savings for the health system (Clark et al., 2013).

It is possible that primary care-led memory clinics are most appropriate where staffing shortages or other capacity constraints lead to long waiting times or otherwise hamper access to specialist services, including specialist memory clinics. In Ontario, at least one family health team closed their memory clinic due to the availability of easily accessible specialist services in their area (Lee et al., 2014). The occasional nature of the memory clinics, which largely operate once or twice per month, and need for minimal additional investments in staff or supplies suggests this model may be well suited to address these resource constraints with minimal disruption to the regular operations of the health system.

In Israel, people with dementia frequently receive care at geriatric clinics, rather than diagnostic memory clinics. Memory clinics are normally specialist-led and primarily located within acute hospitals and other tertiary care facilities. These largely diagnostic memory clinics are outside the public health insurance system, and require pre-approval by insurance funds for visits to be reimbursed. For this reason, most primary care physicians do not refer suspected cases of dementia to diagnostic memory clinics, but rather to in-network geriatric clinics. Often located in the same physical building as the primary care clinic, geriatric clinics are responsible for a range of elderly care services and do not specialise in memory services. Their primary staff includes geriatricians but not psychiatrists or neurologists. While they can conduct diagnostic evaluations for memory disorders, they are less likely to have access to the latest imaging technology and may be less familiar with dementia diagnoses than specialists at dedicated memory clinics. However, as in primary care memory clinics in Canada and the UK, their location in the same building as primary care facilities can help with patient comfort and promotes communication between the person with dementia's primary care physician and the geriatric clinic staff. In an evaluation of geriatric clinics, up to 70% of the patients were found to have been diagnosed with some form of cognitive impairment.

As an alternative to the comprehensive memory clinic, health professionals in a number of countries have developed care clinics that provide post- and sometimes pre-diagnostic support, with the actual diagnostic evaluation conducted elsewhere. In a way, these models build on the expanded notion of a comprehensive memory clinic, by reflecting the understanding that people with dementia may need integrated services that offer signposting and care beyond the clinical diagnosis. In Austria, a model of care management support known as Dementia Service Centres have been developed in the region of Upper Austria (Auer et al., 2015). The centres have three explicit goals: to promote early but timely detection of dementia, to support caregivers, and to delay premature institutionalisation. Recognising that memory clinics and other institutions may have a high physical and psychological barriers for entry, Dementia Service Centres are integrated into the community, encouraging people who may have dementia to be tested at their own pace, and helping them before, during and after the diagnostic process. There are currently eight centres in two regions of the country. The centres respond to a recognised need in Austria, as reflected in the Austrian Dementia Strategy to develop low-threshold centres that support people with dementia and their carers. Initially funded by Austria's national insurance company, the centres are now financed publicly, and will be further rolled out in Upper Austria and possibly other areas of the country in the coming years.

A similar model has been developed in Belgium, where memory rehabilitation centres provide support to people with dementia and their carers, without providing diagnostic services. There are currently 12 memory rehabilitation clinics throughout the country, with at least one located in each province. Clinics are intended to facilitate living in the community longer and offer occupational therapy, home visits, psychoeducation, and support for families. The services of memory rehabilitation centres can be accessed once a person with dementia has received a formal diagnosis of dementia, including from a diagnostic memory clinic. Up to 20 visits to a memory rehabilitation centre are reimbursed over a lifetime.

Memory clinics may be a more appropriate setting for providing care to people with complex cases of dementia, though their cost effectiveness should be considered

The role of memory clinics in providing care beyond diagnosis has become particularly pronounced for complex or uncommon cases of dementia. In some cases, this expanded role has been formalised into guidelines or care pathways for dementia. In Denmark, the extent to which memory clinics are involved in follow-up care depends largely on the case management programmes of each administrative region. In the capital region around Copenhagen, memory clinics are responsible for diagnosis, treatment and follow-up in the first months following diagnosis, after which care management is returned to the primary care physician. Capacity constraints limit the ability of memory clinics to provide longer-term care for all people with dementia. In certain cases, however, including where people with dementia also have special needs or where cases are particularly complex, such as where patients have frontotemporal dementia, memory clinics are expected to offer lifetime follow up care.

Box 2.6. The role of memory clinics in case management: The Healthy Aging Brain Center

The Healthy Aging Brain Center in the US state of Indiana is a memory clinic located in the public health care system 'Wishard Health Services' in Marion County, Indiana. The health system serves a primarily minority, low-income population of about 750 000 in and around the city of Indianapolis. The Healthy Aging Brain Center was launched to improve existing standards of care around diagnosis and management of people with dementia through a model that, while delivered through the Centre, also strengthens the role of primary care physicians, informal carers, and people with dementia. The staff of the Healthy Aging Brain Center includes two geriatricians, two dementia co-ordinators, and one medical assistant (Boustani et al., 2011).

As a diagnostic memory clinic, the Healthy Aging Brain Center (HABC) accepts referrals from general practitioners and specialists, as well as referrals from family members or caregivers and self-referrals. Prior to an initial in-person assessment, a person with possible cognitive impairment and their informal carer will completed a structured needs assessment by phone or mail. If the in-person diagnostic evaluation indicates a diagnosis of dementia, staff at HABC develops a tailored care management plan, the details of which are discussed with the person with dementia and their informal carer at a second in-person meeting. Components of the care plan include pharmacological and non-pharmacological interventions, support and counselling services for the person with dementia and their carers, participation in support groups, telephone support, and the opportunity for co-management in complex cases. In addition, the HABC staff engages in case-finding for other possible comorbidities and behavioural challenges, including depression and psychosis, and actively assesses both the physical and emotional well-being of informal caregivers to monitor carer stress and intervene as needed. Following the initial diagnostic and needs assessment, people with dementia and their carers are followed up by telephone and in-person visits. In-person visits can range from once per month to once per year, based on need.

Compared with people with dementia who received support through primary care centres, people with dementia who accessed the Healthy Aging Brain Center were found to have had fewer and shorter rates of hospitalisation, with lower rates of readmittance and higher health quality outcomes, including better management of high cholesterol (Boustani et al., 2011). The net cost savings from the HABC model have been estimated at up to USD 2 856 per patient, suggesting that substantial cost savings could be generated for health systems if such integrated care models were adopted (French et al., 2014).

Special provisions for complex cases are also made in Norway, where memory clinics are not included in the recommended typical diagnostic pathway. New guidelines released in 2017 advise that in complex and uncommon cases, including cases of early onset dementia, mild cognitive impairment, dementia in people with different language or cultural backgrounds, and dementia accompanied by serious comorbidities, care should be handled by memory clinics. For less complicated cases of dementia, primary care health services, including the general practitioner and municipal memory teams are considered to be sufficient for diagnosis and care. Complex cases are similarly managed by memory clinics in the Netherlands, while most people with less complicated diagnoses of dementia will be referred back to their general practitioner for care following a memory clinic assessment.

While a small number of countries have clearly articulated the expected services offered by memory clinics, in most countries the expansion of services beyond diagnosis has developed in a more ad-hoc manner. A review of memory clinics in Ireland found that of the 14 memory clinics in operation in 2013, 12 specialised in diagnosis, one offered both pre- and post-diagnostic support, one provided post-diagnostic support, and two specialised in caring for people with intellectual disabilities (Cahill et al., 2013). The range of services offered is similarly varied in Austria, Israel, Portugal, and the United States, which lack standards or definitions for memory clinics. In Greece, memory clinics provide diagnostic services and clinical follow-up but do not offer non-pharmacological treatment options or support for families and carers. However, half of memory clinics are located in day care centres associated with the Alzheimer's Association of Greece, ensuring proximity to such services. As in Greece, many memory clinics in Portugal are associated with day care centres and sometimes offer non-pharmacological treatments, including cognitive therapy.

Despite growing interest in memory clinics, their effectiveness – and particularly cost-effectiveness – for diagnosis and care is not clear. A recent study of memory assessment services in the United Kingdom found that while the care provided through memory clinics was effective, it was not cost effective (Gomes et al., 2017). Moreover, whether memory clinics provide more cost-effective post-diagnostic care than primary care settings is far from established. Recent evidence suggests that in many cases, primary care can offer equivalent care for much lower cost. A randomised control trial of follow-up care through memory clinics in the Netherlands found that care provided through memory clinics was no more effective than post-diagnostic support provided through general practitioners (Meeuwsen et al., 2012). There is also evidence that the demographic profile of memory clinic users has changed over time, with memory clinics increasingly seeing people with higher levels of cognitive function (Azam et al., 2016). More evidence is needed to evaluate whether memory clinics are equally effective for people with higher cognitive function, or whether they should be reserved for people with serious cognitive difficulties. Given the cost pressures faced by many health and social care systems, countries should carefully consider whether memory clinics should always be included in the clinical pathway, particularly for post-diagnostic support.

2.3. Efforts must be strengthened to monitor diagnosis rates and improve measurement

In the past years, as dementia has risen on the international policy agenda, many OECD countries have developed or updated their dementia strategies, and there is broad interest in improving the quality of care that people with dementia receive. However, a lack of data on the quality of dementia care continues to hold back improvement efforts. Improving data for dementia is recognised as a key policy in a number of national action and strategic plans, including in Ireland, Switzerland, the UK, and the United States. Other countries have made improving dementia research – not only clinical research, but also population health – a key component of their national plans, including in Australia, Finland, and Mexico. Yet despite these signals, few countries have data systems that can generate the kind of information critical to developing evidence-based policies and measuring progress toward defined goals. Data challenges have further constrained the ability to engage in international comparisons in addition to hampering effective domestic policy development.

In response to this, the OECD recently undertook work to develop a small number of internationally comparable measures of the quality of dementia care. As part of this project, 21 OECD countries participated in a scoping survey aimed at identifying the most promising areas for developing indicators. 14 also participated in a feasibility study. The scoping survey and feasibility study provided important information related to data availability for dementia in OECD countries. An initial set of six pilot indicators was launched in January 2017, with the intention of providing information related to the comparative quality of dementia care across OECD countries.

2.3.1. Few countries have basic data on dementia diagnosis

Diagnosing dementia is critical to responding to dementia and remains a policy priority for many OECD countries. Understanding the success of diagnostic strategies requires an estimate of both the number of people diagnosed with dementia and the total prevalence in the population. Out of 21 reporting countries, 15 can estimate total prevalence at a national level. For the most part, country-level prevalence estimates appear to match estimates in the international literature. More than 70% of countries that submitted prevalence data as part of the 2017 OECD pilot dementia data collection reported prevalence rates that are close to a recent international review of prevalence estimates, which estimated regional prevalence rates based on published prevalence studies (ADI, 2015).

While most countries can estimate dementia prevalence, fewer than 40% of countries can estimate rates of diagnosis nationally. Given the policy priority improving diagnosis rates has received in many countries, establishing a baseline from which to improve is critical. A number of countries, including the United Kingdom (England) and Denmark, have set specific targets around improving diagnosis rates. As part of the Prime Minister's Challenge on Dementia, a target was set to increase dementia diagnosis rates from 42% to two-thirds of people living with dementia in England. In Denmark, the National Action Plan for Dementia has set a goal to increase diagnostic assessment among people living with dementia, including securing a specific diagnosis for 80% of those assessed.

Identifying diagnosed cases of dementia is important to understanding how people with dementia navigate and use health and social care services. Without a dementia diagnosis, people with dementia cannot be tracked through the health system, and any differences in the quality or quantity of care that they might receive cannot be measured. For example, there is compelling evidence indicating that stays in hospital for people with dementia can negatively impact their well-being (Fong et al., 2012; Fick et al., 2013). Reducing both hospital admissions and length of stay in hospital are therefore important policy goals in improving the quality of life of people with dementia. A number of policies in OECD countries have been developed with these outcomes in mind. Without dementia diagnoses recorded consistently in medical records, however, measuring progress and policy effectiveness is not possible. At the moment, less than half of OECD countries can measure the utilisation of health and social care services for people with dementia at a national level (see Figure 2.2.).

Figure 2.2. Countries that can identify people with dementia in administrative data

By care setting (out of 21 OECD countries)

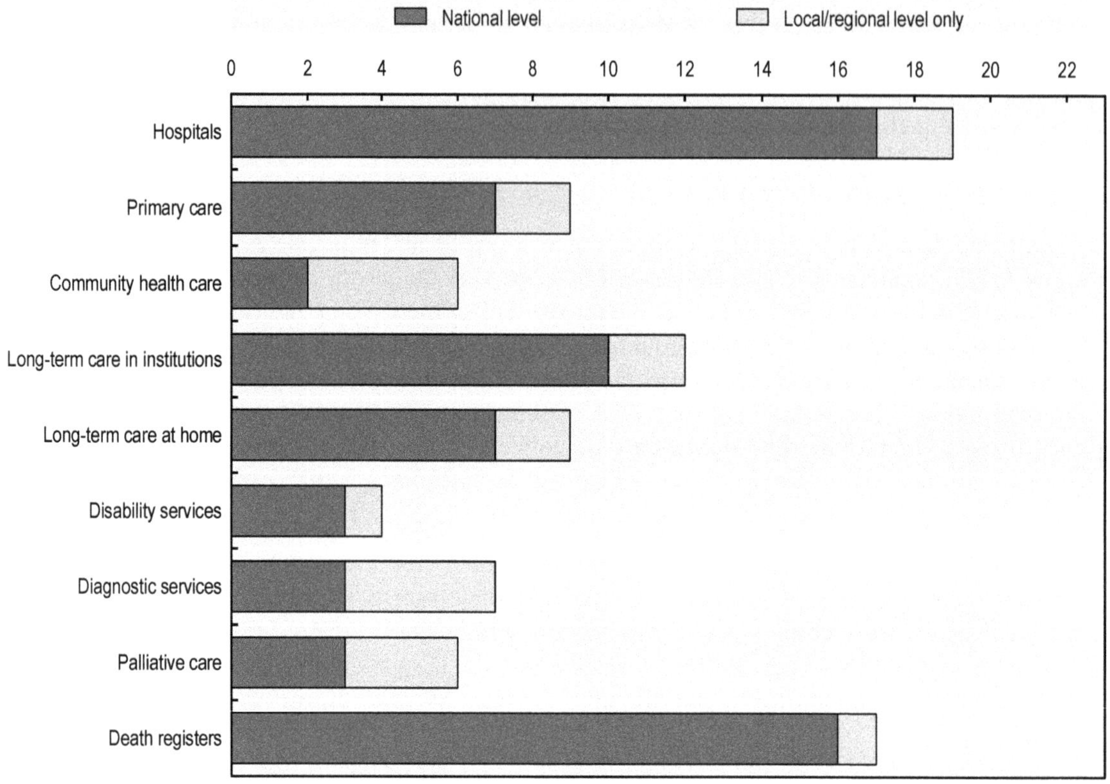

Source: OECD Dementia Care Survey and Interviews 2016-17.

StatLink http://dx.doi.org/10.1787/888933735196

Health data in OECD countries most regularly comes from administrative data (such as insurance datasets), population surveys, patient surveys, clinical records, and disease registries (OECD, 2015b). Many more countries can identify people with dementia in administrative datasets than can do so in registries or surveys. This is in part driven by the fact that administrative datasets are available in all countries. This data is collected to help with the administration of the system – for example, tracking the number and type of patients to determine payments from health insurers to providers – rather than explicitly for research or to measure quality. However, it is possible to derive some information about the quality of care from this type of data. Administrative data also has the advantage that it usually covers all people who interact with a certain part of the system. The most common care setting in which countries use administrative data to identify people with dementia is hospitals. Nearly 80% of surveyed OECD countries can identify people with dementia using national-level administrative hospital data. Data from other care settings is less widely available. Fewer than half of the countries surveyed can identify people with dementia in administrative data from primary care, long-term care (LTC) facilities, LTC provided at home, community health care, disability services, diagnostic services and palliative care.

2.3.2. Effective monitoring of diagnosis rates will require better primary care data or the development of dementia registries

Across the OECD, countries are at very different stages of development in terms of how health data is collected, stored, shared, and used. Countries differ in terms of how data is processed, transferred between organisations, linked across organisations and jurisdictions for federated states, and protected. These different approaches have very real consequences for what is understood about a disease in a country, and how data can be used to maximise health benefits while safeguarding privacy.

Most OECD countries could do more to ensure that primary care data for dementia is accurate. Even where dementia has been diagnosed in primary care, it may not be recorded in patient records. In one study, just 19% of patients who were screened and confirmed to have dementia in Indiana, the United States were found to have a dementia diagnosis subsequently included in their medical records (Boustani et al., 2005). In the UK, coding guidelines for general practitioners were developed through NHS England based on the belief that practitioners may be confused by dementia coding processes (NHS England, 2015).

Even where information about a dementia diagnosis is recorded in primary care data, the information can be difficult to access and share where primary care data is poorly linked to other health data systems. Across the OECD, primary care data remains one of the least regularly linked data sources in the health system. 10 of 22 OECD countries reported that they can link primary care data with other data sources, while just two reported that primary care data is regularly linked with other data sources to monitor health care quality and health systems performance (OECD, 2015b). Eight of 21 OECD countries – Austria, Canada, Finland, France, Latvia, Norway, Spain, and the United Kingdom (Northern Ireland, Scotland, and Wales) reported that primary care administrative datasets that can identify people with dementia were available at the national level. A further four countries – Australia, Japan, the Netherlands, and Sweden – could identify people using registry or survey data.

Dementia registries offer an alternative approach to improving the data landscape. Data registries are increasingly being used by countries to monitor and improve health outcomes related to specific diseases. Across different countries, registries have been shown to improve data transparency and lead to the identification of best practice, better health outcomes, and lower cost of care (Larsson et al., 2012). One study suggested that replicating a hip replacement surgery registry from Sweden could lead to cost savings of 8% in the United States by reducing second surgeries (Larsson et al., 2012). In recent years, a number of countries have developed registries focused specifically on dementia, though they remain uncommon. Six OECD countries have developed dementia registries at either the national or regional level; of those countries with regional dementia registries, at least two are in the process of scaling up to the national level. While dementia registries indicate a concerted effort to improve the data infrastructure for dementia, the depth and coverage of registries differs substantially between countries. A number of major data challenges remain even in the registry model, including incorporating data from different health care settings – notably primary care – and ensuring comprehensive coverage.

Box 2.7. Governing health data: what governance mechanisms are necessary?

In recent years, the OECD has actively participated in global debates considering the key principles that should govern the use of health data. A comprehensive study of national health data systems published in 2015 identified eight key health data governance mechanisms that can help to ensure health data can be used to maximum benefits for patients and societies, while minimising risks to the privacy of patients and to the security of health data:

The health information system supports the monitoring and improvement of health care quality and system performance, as well as research innovations for better health care and outcomes.

The processing and the secondary use of data for public health, research and statistical purposes are permitted, subject to safeguards specified in the legislative framework for data protection.

The public are consulted upon and informed about the collection and processing of personal health data.

A certification or accreditation process for the processing of health data for research and statistics is implemented.

The project approval process is fair and transparent and decision making is supported by an independent, multidisciplinary project review body.

Best practices in data de-identification are applied to protect patient data privacy.

Best practices in data security and management are applied to reduce re-identification and breach risks.

Governance mechanisms are periodically reviewed at an international level to maximise societal benefits and minimise societal risks as new data sources and new technologies are introduced.

Source: OECD (2015), *Health Data Governance: Privacy, Monitoring and Research*, http://dx.doi.org/10.1787/9789264244566-en..

SveDem: The Swedish Dementia Registry

The Swedish Dementia Registry SveDem is arguably the most comprehensive dementia registry currently operating in the OECD. Established in May 2007, the registry includes people receiving new diagnoses of dementia. All people included in the registry receive yearly follow-up. Demographic data, including age and gender and clinical information related to the dementia diagnosis (MMSE score, dementia sub-type, results of the diagnostic evaluation) are both included in the registry. In addition, further information, including pharmacological and non-pharmacological treatments received, available community-based support, and the time it took to receive a formal diagnosis following referral are all recorded (Religa et al., 2015). Separate indicators related to nursing care are also collected when patients reside in a long-term care facility. SveDem has increasingly considered how to incorporate patient-reported measures, including patient-reported outcome measures (PROMs) in their registry. At the moment, only the 'Quality of Life in Late-Stage Dementia' (QUALID) indicator, reported by carers for people with advanced dementia living in nursing homes, is included in the registry. There is recognition that including patient-reported measures for people with dementia in the early stages of the disease would also be beneficial (Religa et al., 2015).

Data is collected from 100% of memory clinics in Sweden, as well as 79% of general practices. Reporting from general practitioners has increased substantially since the launch of the registry, though full coverage may be difficult to achieve. While SveDem offers a useful tool for longitudinal follow-up, it is difficult to encourage general practitioners who see just a small number cases of dementia per year to invest the time it takes to participate in the registry. Sweden currently has 110 distinct disease registries, leading to the possibility that general practitioners may experience 'registry fatigue' and elect not to participate in those that cover conditions where their caseload is low. Nursing homes began to participate in the dementia registry in 2012. The number of nursing homes contributing data has risen from 63 in 2012 to 381 in 2015. Data from hospital settings is not included in the registry. Nursing homes are able to compare statistics from their home to others in the region and across Sweden, offering a useful benchmark for improving quality.

Because SveDem includes data from all memory clinics and the majority of general practices, it is considered a relatively robust measure of dementia incidence in the country. It provides a rich trove of data related both to diagnosis and types and pathways of care following diagnosis. Data from the registry has been used by researchers to further understanding of the dementia care pathway, including analyses of medications treatment by dementia sub-type, diagnostic and treatment differences by gender and age, and cost of diagnosis in primary versus secondary care (Religa et al., 2012; Johnell et al., 2013; Wimo et al., 2013). Seven indicators to measure quality of dementia care have been identified for use from the SveDem data (Religa et al., 2015). These are based on quality indicators identified by the Swedish national guidelines for dementia care and treatment, and are accompanied by target values for the registry to achieve (Religa et al., 2015).

The Danish Dementia Registry

The administrative Capital Region of Denmark initially launched a dementia registry in 2005, covering 30% of the population (Johannsen et al., 2011). The registry, which draws its data from secondary care settings, was expanded to cover the entire country beginning in 2016. Like in Sweden, the Danish registry enrols all new diagnoses of dementia in the database. All 39 memory clinics in Denmark are legally mandated to record new diagnoses of dementia with the registry (Johannsen et al., 2011). Unlike in SveDem, however, general practitioners are not obligated to participate in the registry, limiting the number of diagnoses that may be captured by the system. In Denmark, general practitioners can diagnose dementia, though because medications must be prescribed by a specialist, many dementia patients are likely referred on to specialist care and may still be captured by reporting from memory clinics. Data from nursing homes and inpatient hospital stays are excluded from the registry.

The Danish Dementia Registry was developed as a quality registry, and as such has identified a set of eight process and volume indicators focusing on the evaluative process, as well as target values for each. The Danish indicators were developed with by experts in diagnostic evaluation and are intended to be markers of quality diagnosis that can be easily recorded by clinicians in less than two minutes (Johannsen et al., 2011). In comparison to the Swedish quality indicators, the Danish indicators focus more on the diagnostic process and less on longer-term questions of care. However, the additional information collected by the Danish Dementia Registry, allows for many of the same or similar indicators to be evaluated.

Table 2.5. Quality indicators for dementia care: SveDem and the Danish Dementia Registry

SveDem	Danish Dementia Registry
1. Proportion of patients diagnosed with dementia during last year	1. Percentage of demented patients amongst number of referred
2. Proportion of patients undergoing basic dementia work-up	2. Proportion of patients evaluated within 90 days
3. Proportion of Alzheimer's Disease patients treated with cholinesterase inhibitors and/or memantine	3. Proportion of demented patients assessed with MMSE
	4. Proportion of demented patients assessed with IADL-FAQ scale
4. Proportion of patients treated with antipsychotics in nursing homes	5. Proportion of demented patients with available results of all recommend [sic] blood tests
5. Proportion of patients with day-care at diagnosis	6. Proportion of demented patients with a structural brain scan (CT or MRI)
6. Proportion of patients living in nursing homes\	
7. Proportion of patients followed-up at least once a year	7. Proportion of demented patients where the etiological diagnosis is determined
	8. Proportion of patients with AD, DLB and PDD treated with anti-dementia drugs

Source: Religa et al 2015; Johannsen et al 2011.

Though the Danish Dementia Registry was only rolled out nationwide in 2016, results from the data collected have already been incorporated into dementia policy. Most notably, the results of the 2016 data collection indicated that many of the 39 memory clinics operating in Denmark see very few patients each year. The number of patients evaluated at memory clinics ranged from 5 to 1 200, while a large number of clinics saw fewer than 80 patients in 2016. As a result, as part of the Dementia Action Plan, the government has allocated DKK 170 million (approximately EUR 23 million) to restructuring and improving memory clinics so they are 'bigger, better, and fewer.' Financing will be distributed to the five administrative regions according to how well they meet the recommendations for memory clinics that were recently published by the National Board of Health.

Developing registries from insurance data: examples from Israel and France

SveDem and the Danish Dementia Registry represent a deliberate approach to build a data infrastructure that facilitates the development of a disease-specific registry based on data that was either available and not previously linked, or was not previously collected. In other countries where national insurance systems cover a large part of or close to the entire population, insurance fund data has been used to develop similar dementia registries using information collected for administrative purposes.

In Israel, the third-largest health maintenance organisation, Kupat Holim Meuhedet, developed a methodology to use their administrative data to measure service utilisation for people with dementia. Developed in concert with the Israel Centre for Disease Control, the registry collates dementia diagnoses made at the primary and acute care levels to link patient information across health care settings. In Israel, most diagnoses are made at primary health or geriatric health clinics, both of which are funded by health maintenance organisations. Prescriptions data is also included in the registry, though memory clinics, which are private entities located outside health maintenance organisations, are excluded. The registry will collect information related to health care utilisation in addition to basic demographic information. Initial analyses of the data collected by the dementia registry indicate that people with dementia use more health care resources – including more frequent doctor's visits, more frequent hospitalisations, and longer hospitalisations – than similar populations without dementia. The dementia registry will be rolled out nationally, covering all four health maintenance organisations, by the end of 2017.

As part of the third French National Plan on Alzheimer's Disease and Related disorders (2008-2012), a national dementia registry, the Banque nationale Alzheimer, was launched in 2009. The registry is intended to record all cases of dementia reported by memory clinics and memory research centres in France, as well as cases of dementia diagnosed by independent specialists. As of 2017, 435 memory consultation clinics, 28 memory research centres, and 74 independent specialists have contributed data to the registry, which now includes data on over 800 000 patients across mainland France. Information collected in the registry includes details of the dementia diagnosis, demographic information, and basic information about treatment (both pharmacological and non-pharmacological) and a patient's living circumstances. However, data from other sources – including hospital data, primary care data, and medicines data, is not currently included in the registry. A recent evaluation of the Banque nationale Alzheimer raised questions over the representativeness of people who seek help at memory consultation clinics and memory research centres (Santé publique France, 2017). Among other recommendations, the review strongly encouraged linking the data available in the Banque nationale Alzheimer to other data sources. These include the national health insurance database Sniiram, which could provide information related to medicines consumption, hospitalisation, and registration of a patient with the category affectation de longue durée – a special category of reimbursement open to a limited number of long-term conditions, including dementia. The review additionally recommended linking information in the data bank with the national death registry, CépiDC (Santé publique France, 2017). The Banque nationale Alzheimer is currently undergoing a restructuring to improve the quality of its data and to expand its coverage to allow for a better analysis of care management and the continuum of care experienced by people with dementia.

Dementia surveillance registries in the United States

Three US states – South Carolina, West Virginia, and Georgia – have established databases that link a range of data sources into dedicated dementia registries. First established in 1988, the dementia registry in South Carolina incorporates data from inpatient hospitalisation, Medicaid, mental health records, home health, long-term care evaluations, emergency departments (in South Carolina), state health plans, vital records, community mental health centres and mental health resource centres, and other sources of information linked by a unique patient identifier (UPI) to develop an understanding of the current situation facing the state (Arnold School of Public Health, 2017). While the registry collects information related to the diagnosis, sociodemographic information, caregiver information, and the living circumstances of the person with dementia, it does not collect information on treatments and cannot be seen as a quality register similar to those in Scandinavia.

Dementia registries help to improve dementia care and policy, though in the longer-term countries should strengthen their health data infrastructure

The case studies discussed in this section highlight the range of forms dementia registries have taken across different countries. Other OECD countries have begun to evaluate the usefulness and feasibility of developing dementia registries, with plans for a national registry in Italy and recent calls to develop a registry in Australia. A number of key components can help registries to contribute effectively to our understanding of dementia and the quality of dementia care, and can be used to inform evidence-based policymaking.

Most importantly, dementia registries are most useful when they come close to capturing all diagnosed cases of dementia in a country. The proportion of diagnoses made in different health care settings will differ between countries, but in most of the OECD, both primary care and secondary memory clinics will be important sources of diagnosis. Efforts should be made to include these settings in dementia registries. It may be particularly challenging to include data from primary care clinics, particularly given that dementia likely represents a small proportion of all patients for most primary care physicians. Nevertheless, it is an important source of information, particularly considering that the population visiting their primary care physicians may be more representative of the population than those who continue on to specialised assessment centres. Financial or other incentives could be considered to engage primary care doctors in contributing to the registry. In Sweden, general practitioners were initially paid per diagnostic assessment, to encourage participation, though these benefits have since been lifted. Other important care settings that could be included to improve measuring quality outcomes include nursing homes, acute hospitals, and community-based day care centres.

Data generated from dementia registries can be an important tool in evaluating not only the care received by people with dementia in a given country, but also inform whether the institutions created to facilitate this care are operating as they should be. The reorganisation of memory clinics currently underway in Denmark, as a direct result of the first year of data from the Danish Dementia Registry, suggests that dementia registries are an important source of data in addressing important questions related how the care structures being developed to address dementia can themselves impact the quality of care.

To best facilitate improvements in quality, dementia registries should wherever possible encourage follow-up of individual cases be recorded within the registry. The Swedish BPSD registry provides a good example of how quality of care can be quickly improved when cases are monitored on a regular basis. Ensuring follow-up information is recorded in the registry will allow countries to understand better the full pathway of dementia care. In particular, including data from nursing homes and other intensive care settings would enable countries to use registries to develop a better understanding of living with more advanced forms of the disease.

References

Alzheimer's Disease International (2015), *World Alzheimer Report 2015: The Global Impact of Dementia – An Analysis of Prevalence, Incidence, Cost and Trends*, Alzheimer's Disease International, London.

Arnold School of Public Health, Office for the Study of Aging, University of South Carolina (2017), *2017 Annual Report: South Carolina Alzheimer's Disease Registry*, Columbia: University of South Carolina.

Auer, S. R., Span, E. and B. Reisberg (2015), "Dementia service centres in Austria: A comprehensive support and early detection model for persons with dementia and their caregivers – theoretical foundations and model description", *Dementia*, Vol. 14, No. 4, pp. 513–527. https://doi.org/10.1177/1471301213502214

Azam, B. et al. (2016), "Trends in referred patient profiles in a memory clinic over 20 years", *Dementia*, Vol. 15, No. 4, pp. 789–797. https://doi.org/10.1177/1471301214539691.

Barnes, D. E. et al. (2014), "Development and validation of a brief dementia screening indicator for primary care", *Alzheimer's & Dementia*, Vol. 10, No. 6, pp. 656–665.e1. https://doi.org/10.1016/j.jalz.2013.11.006.

Benbow, S. M. et al. (2013), "Closing the diagnosis gap and improving care: the primary care memory clinic", *Progress in Neurology and Psychiatry*, Vol. 17, No. 6, pp. 27–30.

Borson, S. et al. (2003), "The Mini-Cog as a Screen for Dementia: Validation in a Population-Based Sample", *Journal of the American Geriatrics Society*, Vol. 51,, pp. 1451–1454.

Borson, S. et al. (2007), "Implementing Routine Cognitive Screening of Older Adults in Primary Care: Process and Impact on Physician Behavior", *Journal of General Internal Medicine*, Vol. 22, No. 6, pp. 811–817. https://doi.org/10.1007/s11606-007-0202-8.

Borson, S. et al. (2013), "Improving dementia care: The role of screening and detection of cognitive impairment", *Alzheimer's & Dementia*, Vol. 9, No. 2, pp. 151–159. https://doi.org/10.1016/j.jalz.2012.08.008

Boustani, M. et al. (2005a), "Implementing a screening and diagnosis program for dementia in primary care", *Journal of General Internal Medicine*, Vol. 20, No. 7, pp. 572–577. https://doi.org/10.1007/s11606-005-0103-7

Boustani, M. A. et al. (2011), "Implementing innovative models of dementia care: The Healthy Aging Brain Center", *Aging & Mental Health*, Vol. 15, No. 1, pp. 13–22. https://doi.org/10.1080/13607863.2010.496445

Bradford, A. et al. (2009), "Missed and delayed diagnosis of dementia in primary care: prevalence and contributing factors", *Alzheimer Disease & Associated Disorders*, Vol. 23., No. 4, pp. 306-314.

Cahill, S. and M. Pierce (2013), "Briefing Paper on Dementia Diagnosis", Genio Dementia Series, Briefing Paper No. 3, pp. 1–44, Mulingar, Ireland.

Cheung, G. and J. Strachan (2008), "A Survey of Memory Clinics in New Zealand", *Australasian Psychiatry*, Vol. 16, No. 4, pp. 244–247. https://doi.org/10.1080/10398560701852131

Clark, M. et al. (2013), "Putting personalisation and integration into practice in primary care", *Journal of Integrated Care*, Vol. 21, No. 2, pp. 105–120. https://doi.org/10.1108/14769011311316033.

De Lepeleire, J. et al. (2008), "The primary care diagnosis of dementia in Europe: An analysis using multidisciplinary, multinational expert groups", *Aging & Mental Health*, Vol. 12, No. 5, pp. 568–576. https://doi.org/10.1080/13607860802343043.

Dodd, E. et al. (2014), "An evaluation of primary care led dementia diagnostic services in Bristol", *BMC Health Services Research*, Vol. 14, No. 592, pp. 1–11. https://doi.org/10.1186/s12913-014-0592-3.

Dong, Y. et al. (2010), "The Montreal Cognitive Assessment (MoCA) is superior to the Mini-Mental State Examination (MMSE) for the detection of vascular cognitive impairment after acute stroke", *Journal of the Neurological Sciences*, Vol. 299, No. 1-2, pp. 15–18. https://doi.org/10.1016/j.jns.2010.08.051.

Downs, M. et al. (2006), "Effectiveness of educational interventions in improving detection and management of dementia in primary care: cluster randomised controlled study", *BMJ*, Vol. 332, No. 7543, pp. 692–696. https://doi.org/10.1136/bmj.332.7543.692.

Fick, D. M. et al. (2013), "Delirium superimposed on dementia is associated with prolonged length of stay and poor outcomes in hospitalized older adults", *Journal of Hospital Medicine*, Vol. 8, No. 9, pp. 500–505. https://doi.org/10.1002/jhm.2077.

Fong, T. G. et al. (2012), "Adverse Outcomes After Hospitalization and Delirium in Persons With Alzheimer Disease", *Annals of Internal Medicine*, Vol. 156, No. 12, pp. 848–W296. https://doi.org/10.7326/0003-4819-156-12-201206190-00005.

French, D. D. et al. (2014), "Healthy Aging Brain Center Improved Care Coordination And Produced Net Savings", *Health Affairs*, Vol. 33, No. 4, pp. 613–618. https://doi.org/10.1377/hlthaff.2013.1221

Gomes, M. et al. (2017), "Cost-effectiveness of Memory Assessment Services for the diagnosis and early support of patients with dementia in England", *Journal of Health Services Research & Policy*, Vol. 22, No. 4, pp. 226–235. https://doi.org/10.1177/1355819617714816.

Greaves, I. et al. (2015), "Gnosall Primary Care Memory Clinic: Eldercare facilitator role description and development", *Dementia*, Vol. 14, No. 4, pp. 389–408. https://doi.org/10.1177/1471301213497737

Guideline Adaptation Committee (2016), *Clinical Practice Guidelines and Principles of Care for People with Dementia*, Guideline Adaptation Committee, National Health and Medical Research Council, Sydney.

Hughes, C. (2011), "What you need to know about the Medicare Preventive Services Expansion", *Family Practice Management*, January/February, pp. 22–25.

Johannsen, P. et al. (2011), "Development of a dementia assessment quality database", *Aging & Mental Health*, Vol. 15, No. 1, pp. 40–46. https://doi.org/10.1080/13607863.2010.508769

Johnell, K., Religa, D. and M. Eriksdotter (2013), "Differences in drug therapy between dementia disorders in the Swedish Dementia Registry: A nationwide study of over 7,000 patients", *Dementia and Geriatric Cognitive Disorders*, Vol. 35, pp. 239-248. https://doi.org/10.1159/000348408.

Jolley, D., Benbow, S. M. and M. Grizzell (2006), "Memory clinics", *Postgraduate Medical Journal*, Vol. 82, No. 965, pp. 199–206. https://doi.org/10.1136/pgmj.2005.040592

Khanassov, V., Vedel, I. and P. Pluye (2014), "Barriers to Implementation of Case Management for Patients With Dementia: A Systematic Mixed Studies Review", *The Annals of Family Medicine*, Vol. 12, No. 5, pp. 456–465. https://doi.org/10.1370/afm.1677

Larsson, S. et al. (2012), "Use Of 13 Disease Registries In 5 Countries Demonstrates The Potential To Use Outcome Data To Improve Health Care's Value", *Health Affairs*, Vol. 31, No. 1, pp. 220–227. https://doi.org/10.1377/hlthaff.2011.0762

Lathren, C. R. et al. (2013), "Improving dementia diagnosis and management in primary care: a cohort study of the impact of a training and support program on physician competency, practice patterns, and community linkages", *BMC Geriatrics*, Vol. 13, No. 134.

Le Couteur, D.G. et al. (2013), "Political drive to screen for pre-dementia: not evidence based and ignores the harms of diagnosis", *BMJ*, Vol. 347: f5125. doi https://doi.org/10.1136/bmj.f5125.

Lee, L. et al. (2014), "Primary Care–Based Memory Clinics: Expanding Capacity for Dementia Care", *Canadian Journal on Aging*, Vol. 33, No. 3, pp. 307–319. https://doi.org/10.1017/S0714980814000233.

Lee, L., Kasperski, M.J. and W.W. Weston (2011), "Building capacity for dementia care", *Canadian Family Physician*, Vol. 57,, pp. e249–e252.

Lindesay, J. et al. (2002), "The second Leicester survey of memory clinics in the British Isles", *International Journal of Geriatric Psychiatry*, Vol. 17, No. 1, pp. 41–47. https://doi.org/10.1002/gps.522.

Livingston, G. et al. (2017), "Dementia prevention, intervention, and care", *The Lancet*, Vol. 390, No. 10113, pp. 1–62. https://doi.org/10.1016/S0140-6736(17)31363-6.

Mate, K. E. et al. (2017), "An evaluation of the additional benefit of population screening for dementia beyond a passive case-finding approach", *International Journal of Geriatric Psychiatry*, Vol. 32, No. 3, pp. 316–323. https://doi.org/10.1002/gps.4466.

Meeuwsen, E. J. et al. (2012), "Effectiveness of dementia follow-up care by memory clinics or general practitioners: randomised controlled trial", *BMJ*, Vol. 344,, pp. e3086. https://doi.org/10.1136/bmj.e3086.

Mitchell, A. J., Meader, N. and M. Pentzek (2011), "Clinical recognition of dementia and cognitive impairment in primary care: a meta-analysis of physician accuracy", *Acta Psychiatrica Scandinavica*, Vol. 124, No. 3, pp. 165–183. https://doi.org/10.1111/j.1600-0447.2011.01730.x

Nakanishi, M., and T. Nakashima (2014), "Features of the Japanese national dementia strategy in comparison with international dementia policies: How should a national dementia policy interact with the public health- and social-care systems?", *Alzheimer's & Dementia*, Vol. 10, No. 4, pp. 468-476. http://dx.doi.org/10.1016/j.jalz.2013.06.005.

Nasreddine, Z. S. et al. (2005), "The Montreal Cognitive Assessment, MoCA: a Brief Screening Tool for Mild Cognitive Impairment", *Journal of the American Geriatrics Society*, Vol. 53, No. 4, pp. 695–699.

National Institute for Health & Care Excellence (NICE) (2006), *Dementia: supporting people with dementia and their carers in health and social care: Clinical Guideline*, http://nice.org.uk/guidance/cg42.

NHS England (2015), *Dementia diagnosis and management: A brief pragmatic resource for general practitioners*, NHS England, Publications Gateway Reference Number 02615.

OECD (2015b), *Health Data Governance: Privacy, Monitoring and Research*, OECD Health Policy Studies, OECD Publishing, Paris, http://dx.doi.org/10.1787/9789264244566-en.

OECD (2015a), *OECD Reviews of Health Care Quality: Japan 2015: Raising Standards*, OECD Reviews of Health Care Quality, OECD Publishing, Paris, http://dx.doi.org/10.1787/9789264225817-en.

OECD (2017), *Health at a Glance 2017: OECD Indicators*, OECD Publishing, Paris, http://dx.doi.org/10.1787/health_glance-2017-en.

Religa D. et al. (2012), "Dementia Diagnosis Differs in Men and Women and Depends on Age and Dementia Severity: Data from SveDem, the Swedish Dementia Quality Registry", *Dementia and Geriatric Cognitive Disorders*, Vol. 33, pp. 90–95.

Religa, D. et al. (2015), "SveDem, the Swedish Dementia Registry – A Tool for Improving the Quality of Diagnostics, Treatment and Care of Dementia Patients in Clinical Practice", *PLoS ONE*, Vol. 10, No. 2, pp. e0116538–14. https://doi.org/10.1371/journal.pone.0116538.

Robinson, L., Tang, E., and J.P. Taylor (2015), "Dementia: timely diagnosis and early intervention", *BMJ*, Vol. 350, No. 14, pp. h3029–h3029. https://doi.org/10.1136/bmj.h3029

Santé publique France (2017), "La banque nationale Alzheimer, un outil pour la surveillance épidémiologique des démences en France ?" Santé publique France.

Tannebæk, K. et al. (2014), "The Danish ABC dementia: new e-learning for professional caregivers", *Alzheimer's & Dementia*, Vol. 10,, pp. P180–P181. https://doi.org/10.1016/j.jalz.2014.04.200

Turner, J. J. (2013), "Proposed model of early dementia screening cannot be valid", *BMJ*, Vol. 346, No. 1, pp. f505–f505. https://doi.org/10.1136/bmj.f505

Trzepacz, P. T. et al. (2015), "Relationship between the Montreal Cognitive Assessment and Mini-mental State Examination for assessment of mild cognitive impairment in older adults", *BMC Geriatrics*, Vol. 15, No. 107, pp. 1–9. https://doi.org/10.1186/s12877-015-0103-3.

Tsolaki, M. et al. (2010). "Consensus statement on dementia education and training in Europe", The *Journal of Nutrition, Health & Aging*, Vol. 14, No. 2, pp. 131-135.

UK National Screening Committee (2015), "UK NSC dementia screening recommendation", https://legacyscreening.phe.org.uk/dementia.

U.S. Preventive Services Task Force (2014), "Understanding Task Force Recommendations: Screening for cognitive impairment in older adults", Task Force Final Recommendation.

Waldorff, F.B. and S. Moller (2001), "Diagnostic evaluation of dementia in general practice in Denmark. A national survey", *Scandinavian Journal of Primary Health Care*, Vol. 19, No. 2, pp. 117–121. https://doi.org/10.1080/028134301750235367.

Waldorff, F.B. et al. (2003), "Implementation of a clinical dementia guideline", *Scandinavian Journal of Primary Health Care*, Vol. 21, No. 3, pp. 142-147. https://doi.org/10.1080/02813430310005136.

Wimo, A. et al. (2013), "Costs of diagnosing dementia: results from SveDem, the Swedish Dementia Registry", *International Journal of Geriatric Psychiatry*, Vol. 28, No. 10, pp. 1039–1044. https://doi.org/10.1002/gps.3925

Woodward, M. C. and E. Woodward (2009), "A national survey of memory clinics in Australia", *International Psychogeriatrics*, Vol. 21, No. 4, pp. 696–702. https://doi.org/10.1017/S1041610209009156.

Zadikoff, C. et al. (2008), "A comparison of the mini mental state exam to the Montreal cognitive assessment in identifying cognitive deficits in Parkinson's disease", *Movement Disorders*, Vol. 23, No. 2, pp. 297–299. https://doi.org/10.1002/mds.21837.

Annex 2.A. Primary care in OECD countries

Annex Table 2.A.1. Summary of the role of primary care in OECD countries

Australia	General Practitioners are the entry point to the health system and may administer basic cognitive assessments. These could include the MMSE or other assessments developed for particular population groups and blood tests. Australias Clinical Practice Guidelines and Principles of Care for People with Dementia currently recommend that people with a possible diagnosis of dementia should be referred to memory assessment specialists or services for a formal diagnosis
Austria	General practitioners administer basic cognitive assessments, most commonly the MMSE, and can give a general but not specialised diagnosis. They cannot initiate anti-dementia medications. Most primary care physicians refer suspected cases of dementia on to specialists.
Belgium	There is no diagnostic pathway at the primary level for diagnosing dementia. Primary care physicians administer basic assessments (the MMSE, blood tests) and refer suspected cases on to specialist assessment. They can give a general but not specialised diagnosis. Primary care physicians cannot prescribe anti-dementia medications.
Canada	Provinces are responsible for health care in Canada, and different provinces have developed different clinical pathways and plans around diagnosis and care for dementia. In many of these cases, primary care serves a prominent role. In British Columbia, for example, primary care physicians may diagnose dementia, and integrated primary and community care is seen as a critical base for health service delivery. Similarly, the dementia plan of Alberta includes as a main outcome that Albertans living with dementia and their caregivers receive timely recognition, diagnosis and clinical management *through primary health care*, supported by specialized services (The Provincial Dementia Action Plan for British Columbia 2012; Alberta Dementia Strategy and Action Plan 2017).
Chile	Primary care physicians are the focal point for dementia diagnosis in Chile. They conduct basic assessments (most commonly the MMSE) and can both diagnose dementia and prescribe anti-dementia medications.
Czech Republic	Primary care physicians can do basic assessment, but do not serve as gatekeepers to specialist services. Where there is a suspicion of dementia, primary care physicians most often refer patients to specialists for formal diagnosis. Only specialists can prescribe anti-dementia medications.
Denmark	Primary care physicians, along with dementia co-ordinators, serve as the point of entry into health services for dementia. Primary care physicians perform blood tests and basic assessment tests, such as the MMSE. While they can formally diagnose dementia, prescriptions require a specialist diagnosis. An instrument to help primary care physicians in conducting diagnostic evaluations is under development as part of the 2017-2019 national plan.
Estonia	Primary care physicians serve as a partial gatekeeper to specialist services: referrals are required for neurology but not psychiatry. Clinical guidelines recommend the MMSE assessment. While they can diagnose dementia, primary care physicians most often refer suspected cases on to specialists for formal diagnosis. They cannot prescribe anti-dementia medications.
France	The general practitioner normally serves as the first point of contact when people are concerned about symptoms of dementia. Following an initial clinical exam and interview, general practitioners will refer the patient to a specialist or specialised team neurologists, geriatricians, psychiatrists or a memory consultation team for further testing.
Finland	Primary care physicians are the first point of entry into the health care system for people with dementia, and conduct basic lab and assessment tests, including blood tests, hormonal and thyroid testing, and the MMSE or similar. They can neither formally diagnose nor prescribe anti-dementia medications.
Greece	Primary care physicians play only a minor role in dementia care in Greece. Most people with memory problems go straight to specialist care.
Hungary	Primary care physicians most frequently assess people with suspicion of cognitive impairment with a basic clock test and interview. The MMSE and other assessments are infrequently used. Patients are sometimes referred on to specialists for further diagnostic assessment.
Mexico	Primary care physicians serve as the main point of diagnosis and care for people with dementia in Mexico. They can diagnose dementia, but not prescribe anti-dementia medications. The MMSE exam and geriatric depression scale are most frequently used to assess cognitive impairment and symptoms of dementia.
Netherlands	Primary care physicians are always the gatekeeper to further specialist care in the Netherlands. Initial cognitive impairment is assessed through the MMSE exam, the clock test, and a discussion with the patient and their family members. GPs can both diagnose dementia and prescribe anti-dementia medications, though patients are frequently referred onward to specialists for a more specific diagnosis.

New Zealand	While there is no formal guideline for dementia care at the primary level, most primary care physicians only refer complex cases to specialists, managing non-complex cases at the primary level. No specific tools are specified for diagnosis, though short assessments, including MOCA and MMSE, as well as blood tests, are normally used. Some district health boards (DHBs) now also advise primary care physicians to prescribe CT scans as part of a dementia diagnosis. Primary care physicians can both diagnose dementia and prescribe anti-dementia medications.
Norway	Norwegian guidelines recommend that people with possible dementia should be assessed by both primary health teams and specialist memory clinics. Primary care physicians have access to a template of assessment tools, and nearly always assess cognitive impairment using the MMSE, clock test, and an assessment of activities of daily living (ADL) function.
Portugal	Most diagnosis occurs through specialist assessment. Primary care physicians regularly carry out the MMSE and clock test before referring patients on to specialist care. They cannot prescribe anti-dementia medications.
Slovak Republic	Primary care physicians always serve as the gatekeeper to the health system. They cannot diagnose dementia or prescribe anti-dementia drugs. Prior to referring people with possible dementia to specialists, primary care physicians usually administer the MMSE assessment. The government is working to expand use of the clock test and Montreal Cognitive Assessment (MOCA).
Slovenia	Primary care physicians have no official guidance on detecting and managing dementia. They can neither formally diagnose nor prescribe anti-dementia medications.
Sweden	Primary care physicians can formally diagnose dementia and prescribe anti-dementia drugs for non-complex cases. Assessment at the primary level includes the MMSE cognitive assessment, blood tests, and a CT scan.
Switzerland	Physicians in primary care can both formally diagnose and prescribe anti-dementia medications. Assessment tools used include the MMSE, MOCA, DemTech, and clock test.
Turkey	Primary care physicians cannot diagnose dementia or prescribe anti-dementia drugs. Assessment for dementia always occurs in a hospital clinic.
United Kingdom	Primary care physicians most commonly serve as the first point of contact for persons with memory complaints. They typically conduct a simple memory test and order standard blood tests to rule out other causes of memory problems. General practitioners would normally refer suspected cases of dementia to a memory clinic, memory assessment service, an old age psychiatry community mental health team, or neurologist for further testing and an official diagnosis. Increasingly, a small proportion of people are receiving a diagnosis directly in primary care.
United States	Primary care physicians play a role in cognitive screening as part of the Medicare Annual Wellness Visit. Most assessments of cognitive impairment include short cognitive assessments (mini cog, MOCA) and blood tests.

Source: OECD Dementia Survey and Interviews 2016-2017.

Chapter 3. Helping people with dementia live well in the community

This chapter reviews how countries are enabling people with dementia to live in their communities independently. It assesses what countries are doing to improve co-ordination and access to care and services following a diagnosis, what they have done to make their communities more dementia-friendly, and how informal carers of people with dementia are supported in their role. While there is a growing body of good practice for community-based care, care co-ordination, dementia-friendly initiatives and support for informal carers must be better developed and more regularly measured to further progress.

The statistical data for Israel are supplied by and under the responsibility of the relevant Israeli authorities. The use of such data by the OECD is without prejudice to the status of the Golan Heights, East Jerusalem and Israeli settlements in the West Bank under the terms of international law.

3.1. Meeting the needs of people with dementia at home

In recent years, OECD countries have begun to encourage ageing at home for as long as possible. Many elderly people, including those with dementia, wish to remain in their communities for as long as possible. Because loneliness can accelerate the progression of dementia, it is particularly important that people with dementia avoid social isolation and maintain their relationships for as long as possible. Living at home allows people with dementia to stay independent and connected to their communities.

People with dementia have specific needs that must be met to age at home. Staying at home can pose unique challenges as the disease progresses and symptoms such as wandering increase. Once-familiar home environments can become difficult and even hazardous to navigate, and can contribute to accidents, such as falls. Assistive technologies, such as location tracking devices and automatic reminders, can help people with daily activities. Even where such technologies are available, however, uptake is not always high. Moreover, community services and activities may be underprepared to accommodate people living with dementia.

Many countries have moved in recent years to support this preference and increasingly promote community care and delaying institutionalisation for as long as possible. Delaying onset into residential care and improving community living for people with dementia has been a major policy goal in many countries, and is mentioned in national strategies and plans in Australia, Ireland, Japan, Norway, Sweden, and the United Kingdom, among other OECD countries.

As community-based care is increasingly promoted, some countries with well-established long-term care services have reduced residential long-term care capacity. Between 2005 and 2015, Sweden reduced the number of long-term care beds in institutions by 23.5 beds per 1000 population over aged 65. These reductions can be attributed to a concerted effort to move long-term care out of residential facilities and into the community (Colombo et al., 2011). Other countries, including Australia, Japan, the Netherlands, Denmark, and Norway have also significantly reduced the number of beds per 1 000 people aged 65 and over available in long-term care (Figure 3.1).

Figure 3.1. Trends in long-term beds in institutions and hospitals, 2005-15

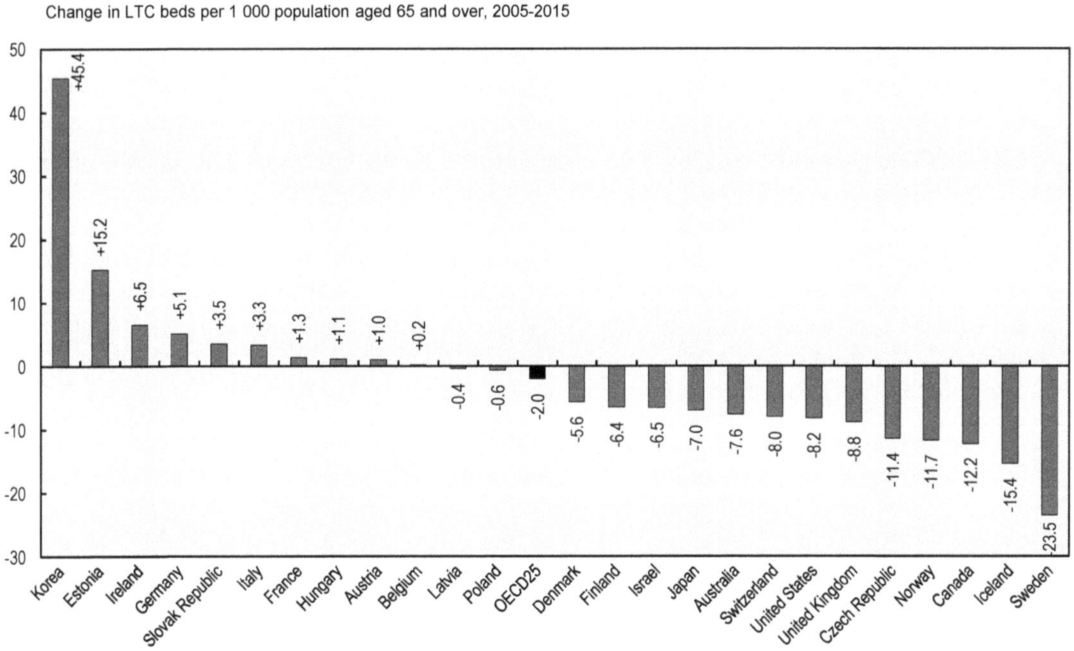

Source: *OECD Health Statistics 2017*, http://dx.doi.org/10.1787/health-data-en.

StatLink http://dx.doi.org/10.1787/888933735215

Providing community-based care to people with dementia can be less efficient than institutional alternatives. Home care aides must travel to individual homes and can care for fewer people than in a residential home, while economies of scale available in institutional care settings are not realised when care is delivered in the community. Informal carers must also provide more hours of care than they would for people in nursing homes. However, community-based care can be substantially cheaper for governments. Cost-saving for public budgets can be realised through reductions in expenditure on board and care in institutions, while the cost of informal care is nearly always excluded from estimates of the cost of care, despite its important contribution.

3.1.1. Services for people diagnosed with dementia

Medications remain the most widely available treatment option and can slow the progress of dementia

While there is no cure for dementia, a number of available medications have been found to have mild effects on cognition for people with certain dementia sub-types and are frequently initiated following a diagnosis. These include memantine, which is applicable for people with Alzheimer's dementia, dementia with Lewy bodies, and Parkinson's disease, and anti-cholinesterase inhibitors, including donepezil, reivastigmine, and galantamine. Both memantine and anti-cholinesterase inhibitors have been found by meta-analyses to have small but beneficial effects on cognition (Livingston et al., 2017). Memantine has been suggested to have a small effect on cognition for people with moderate to severe Alzheimer's disease, while anti-cholinesterase inhibitors have been found to be beneficial for people with Parkinson's with dementia and possibly for dementia with Lewy bodies (McShane et al., 2006; Rolinski et al., 2012). The differing performance of memantine and anti-cholinesterase inhibitors points to the importance of conducting a full diagnostic evaluation and identifying the dementia sub-type wherever possible.

Anti-dementia medications are largely reimbursed across OECD countries. All European OECD members except Latvia at least partially reimburse either donepezil, rivastigmine, or galantamine (Alzheimer Europe, 2017). Generic versions of all anti-dementia medications are available. Some countries do not reimburse memantine, though in these cases at least one anti-cholinesterase inhibitor is available (Alzheimer's Europe, 2017). Despite an increasing focus on delivering care through general practitioners, most countries continue to require a specialist diagnosis for a prescription to be initiated. Considering that anti-dementia medications work differently based on dementia sub-type, and that most full diagnostic evaluations are conducted at the specialist level, this restriction may be effective in avoiding inappropriate medicines prescribing.

At the same time, a perceived lack of treatment options is a major barrier to encouraging primary care physicians to diagnose dementia, or to refer patients for further evaluation, suggesting that expanding prescribing rights to primary care physicians could be one approach to increasing assessment, diagnosis and care at the primary level. In a limited number of countries, primary care physicians and sometimes even non-physician health professionals are also allowed to prescribe anti-dementia medications. General practitioners are able to prescribe these medications in Sweden and Denmark, while in the Netherlands, nurses are also allowed to prescribe medications for people with dementia.

Data from countries with dementia registries suggests that a high proportion of people who have received a dementia diagnosis are prescribed at least one anti-dementia medication. In both Sweden and Denmark, more than 80% of patients with Alzheimer's disease, dementia with Lewy bodies, and Parkinson's disease with dementia are treated with medications, with 83% of patients in Sweden and 86% of patients in Denmark receiving anti-dementia drugs (Fereshtehnejad et al., 2014). Though treatment levels are very high, at least one country is reconsidering its support for these medications. France recently launched an inquiry into anti-dementia medications and is evaluating whether or not to continue reimbursing them for people with dementia, citing possible insufficient effectiveness.

A range of non-pharmacological treatments are available in OECD countries

In addition to limited medications available to treat dementia, a number of non-pharmacological interventions have been developed. While pharmacological treatments have focused on improving cognition or delaying further deterioration, most non-pharmacological interventions focus on improving the quality of life for persons living with dementia or their carers. Non-pharmacological interventions proposed for dementia include multi-sensory stimulation, art, music and dance therapies, animal therapy, exercise therapy, reminiscence therapy, massage, and cognitive stimulation therapy. The evidence to support non-pharmacological interventions in improving memory or delaying cognitive deterioration is weak (Kane et al., 2017).

Cognitive stimulation therapy aims to improve cognition through engaging in cognitive activities, including reminiscence therapy and multi-sensory stimulation (Aguirre et al., 2013). A structured programme of CST has been developed and tested in randomized control trials, comprising seven weeks of twice-weekly group sessions for people with early to mild dementia. A Cochrane review of 15 randomised control trials evaluating cognitive stimulation found that the effect of CST on cognition may be equivalent to or better than the impact of anti-cholinesterase inhibitors (Woods et al., 2012). The longer-term effects of cognitive stimulation therapy are less well understood, though there is evidence that engaging in a weekly 'maintenance' session following the initial seven weeks sustained the benefits of the initial CST programme for at least a limited time (Orrell et al., 2005). Maintenance cognitive stimulation therapy has been found to be particularly effective, and also cost-effective, when combined with anti-cholinesterase inhibitors (D'Amico et al., 2015). Cognitive stimulation therapy (CST) is the only non-pharmacological intervention that has been recommended by the UK's National Institute for Health and Care Excellence (NICE) for dementia care and has been found to be cost effective in treating people with dementia (National Collaborating Centre for Mental Health, 2016). It is offered widely in the UK, where about one-third of community mental health services offer group CST, and is available in at least some locations in other OECD countries, including Australia, Canada, Chile, Germany, Israel, Italy, Japan, the Netherlands, New Zealand, Portugal, Korea, and the United States (International Cognitive Stimulation Therapy Centre, UCL, 2017, Orrell et al., 2012).

There is substantial evidence indicating that exercise has a protective role in reducing the risk of developing dementia (Larson et al., 2006; Andel et al., 2008). A number of studies further suggest that exercise may also have a protective factor in cognition, even after the onset of mild cognitive impairment (Lautenschlager et al., 2008). While a Cochrane review of exercise studies found that there was no evidence to indicate that exercise interventions affects cognition or neuropsychiatric symptoms of dementia, there is some evidence to suggest that exercise interventions above a certain level of intensity may help to attenuate cognitive decline in at least mild Alzheimer's disease, suggesting that meta-analyses examining multiple interventions may find no effect because of the differing intensities of different interventions (Forbes et al., 2015; Hoffman et al., 2016). Exercise interventions have further been found to improve performance of activities of daily living (ADL) in people with dementia (Forbes et al., 2015, Öhman et al., 2016). While the overall evidence supporting exercise interventions on cognitive decline is mixed, its overall benefits to health and impacts on activities of daily living, and the relatively low threshold to engage in at least low-intensity exercise activities, indicate that exercise programmes for people living with dementia should be encouraged.

Exercise-related activities are offered in many countries, often through community-based day care and other activity centres. Chile's Kintun day care centre model promotes engaging in physical activity, including playing soccer with local youth. In New Zealand, Alzheimer's Auckland runs a weekly gym group for local community-dwelling people living with dementia (New Zealand Framework for Dementia Care, 2013). Similar community-based exercise initiatives are widely available to people living with dementia in Australia, including targeted exercise activities offered through a community Dementia Gym and exercise activities designed specifically for people with early onset dementia (Alzheimer's Australia, 2014).

Although most non-pharmacological treatments do not appear to alter the progress of dementia, they can play an important role in improving quality of life

Even where non-pharmacological interventions do not show an effect on cognition, they should be considered for the impact they can have on quality of life. So long as no cure for dementia exists, policies for people with dementia and their families and carers should equally consider how different programmes can affect their quality of life. This expanded conception of care beyond the clinical can challenge both health and social systems, where limited resources necessitate decision-making based on clinical outcomes and cost effectiveness. The range of quality of life measures developed for dementia, and recent emphasis on better incorporating patient- and carer-reported measures, is an encouraging step.

A range of alternative non-pharmacological interventions are regularly offered to people living with dementia, including arts- and music-based interventions. These interventions do not appear to have significant effects on cognitive decline, and the quality of current evidence is poor. However, arts-based therapies have been demonstrated to reduce depression and agitation among people living with dementia and improve their overall quality of life, as reported using carer- and patient-reported measures. Music, dance, and art therapies are regularly made available through community day centres, Alzheimer's Associations, and local organisations. In Japan, art therapy and music programmes are made available to people living with dementia who attend community day care centres covered by care insurance (Suzuki et al., 2004). In the United States, the Alzheimer's Association has developed a fine arts programme, Memories in the Making, intended to improve quality of life among people with early or moderate dementia through encouraging self-expression through art. Originally started in Cincinnati, Ohio, the programme has since spread to chapters of the Alzheimer's Association throughout the United States. Because such programmes are largely organised by non-profit organisations and are not part of official care pathways for dementia, information related to their coverage and reach is in most cases limited.

The evidence base supporting most non-pharmacological treatments has largely comprised of short-term evaluations focused on different aspects related to quality of life or reductions in depression and agitation. The different methods of evaluating quality of life has made comparing the findings between studies difficult and points to the importance of developing strong measures of patient-reported measures that can be used across research settings. There is much more limited evidence related to the effects of non-pharmacological interventions on cognition, though some evidence to suggest that cognitive and exercise interventions may have a limited impact on cognition.

As discussed above, a range of non-pharmacological treatments have been found to improve quality of life measures for people living with dementia or their carers, even in the absence of cognitive improvement. These programmes, including exercise therapies, arts-based therapies, and other social group activities, should be made available to people with dementia wherever possible, either through government-funded day centres or non-profit institutions. At the very least, such activities promote social contact and can help to prevent isolation and loneliness in people with dementia.

Measuring treatment is complicated by data constraints

Despite the availability of treatment options that can improve cognition and function in people with dementia, many countries do not have a good picture of how many people receive these services. 11 of 21 OECD countries reported that they could monitor the utilisation of health and social care services for people with dementia at a national level, with a further two (Ireland and Switzerland) reporting that it was possible for at least some regions. Where medications are reimbursed, countries can often record whether a person diagnosed with dementia has received anti-dementia drugs. Systems to track medications consumption are available in many countries, including Canada, Denmark, Finland (through the Social Security Institute), France, Ireland, Israel, Norway, Sweden, and the United Kingdom. However, without comprehensive data about the total number of people diagnosed with dementia, monitoring the *proportion* of people diagnosed with dementia who receive medications is more complex. Countries with comprehensive dementia registries (such as Denmark and Sweden) or those that have more linked health data systems (such as the United Kingdom) can use their data on diagnoses and medications consumption to monitor access to medicines among people with dementia.

3.2. Ensuring adequate access to care after diagnosis

3.2.1. Care co-ordination can help people to access the services they need after a diagnosis

Despite increasing focus on strengthening post-diagnostic support, in most countries, care following diagnosis remains highly fragmented and largely ad-hoc for people with dementia. Though many health and social care services exist that can help people with dementia and their families living in the community, navigating these services can be difficult. People may not know what services are available, or how to access them. Coordinated post-diagnostic support, such as care co-ordination pathways or case management, can help people take advantage of the best support possible.

The organisation of services available to people with dementia and their carers is structured differently between and often within countries. In some cases, a formal diagnosis of dementia is an important eligibility criteria for accessing additional health and social services. How these care services are organised in the health and social systems can broadly be defined as ***care co-ordination***. Sometimes, people with dementia are connected with an individual or group of individuals to help them navigate and access available care services. These more personalised services –which are sometimes a formalised care pathway, and sometimes more ad-hoc – can be considered types of ***case management***.

Most OECD countries have recognised that even where diagnostic pathways are relatively strong, there is substantial room for improvement in strengthening post-diagnostic support for people with dementia and their families. Strengthening access to care and support following a dementia diagnosis is a key policy goal in many national plans. In Australia, improving access to post-diagnostic support and ongoing care and support are priority actions of the 2015-2019 National Framework for Action on Dementia, while in Austria, developing "consistent framework conditions for coordinated care" is one of seven key goals of the 2015 Dementia Strategy. Implementing a chain of care that encourages co-ordination is similarly a goal of in Switzerland's federal strategy, while implementing a system of continuing coordinated care is one of nine objectives articulated in Chile's national plan for dementia.

Despite widespread recognition of the need to improve care co-ordination following diagnosis and more generally along the care pathway, what constitutes care co-ordination, and how it is practiced, differs widely within the OECD. Care co-ordination programmes in OECD countries can be broadly defined in four categories. Where countries lack formalised care co-ordination structures for patients with dementia or other conditions, care co-ordination available is done on a more ad-hoc basis. A number of countries have developed care co-ordination or case management pathways that are implemented in health and social care systems for all people with an eligible condition, and are not limited to or tailored towards people living with dementia. Others offer care co-ordination opportunities that are tailored specifically for dementia. Lastly, some countries offer dementia-specific care co-ordination and case management programmes that are limited to a specific subset of the broader dementia population, with eligibility often determined by the severity or complexity of the case.

Local and ad-hoc initiatives make up for co-ordination services where none are available

A large number of OECD countries, particularly in Eastern Europe and Latin America, report having no care co-ordination services organised for people with dementia to help them navigate social and health services following a diagnosis of dementia. Though strengthening co-ordination of care and case management is a major goal of Chile's dementia strategy, there is currently little support for people with dementia living in the community. In the absence of case management, the state is developing the role of a 'community manager' to make home visits to people with dementia. While the community manager supports people with dementia directly through home visits, they will also engage in case finding and act as an advocate for people with dementia in the community, raising awareness and understanding for the condition.

In a number of countries where neither care co-ordination nor case management is institutionalised, primary care clinics and physicians sometimes provide support to their patients. In Mexico, a limited number of primary care clinics offer some case management to their patients. Similarly, in Hungary and Slovenia people with dementia do not receive care co-ordination in a formalised way, though some experienced general practitioners will connect their patients with relevant services through their network of colleagues in the local area. In Switzerland, general practitioners and memory clinics sometimes organise roundtables, inviting the person with dementia, their family, physicians, and sometimes a social worker to discuss the diagnosis and next steps. Overall, however, co-ordination is seen to be very weak in Switzerland, with no organised care co-ordination available for people with dementia. A 2017 report commissioned by the federal government to review the state of care co-ordination for people with dementia found that just 10% of experts believed that care co-ordination and providing people with dementia with necessary information works well today (Bundesamtes für Gesundheit, 2017). The government recently published recommendations for strengthening care co-ordination, a major goal of Switzerland's federal dementia strategy (Bundesamtes für Gesundheit, 2017).

Case management services are sometimes integrated into memory clinics and other dementia specialist care. In England, case management is generally available for anyone seen in a memory clinic. Case managers are typically allocated based on the severity of the condition and complexity of needs, and often receive specialist training for the position.

In some systems where no institutionalised care co-ordination has been developed, local initiatives have developed support programmes creating local care pathways for people with dementia. With funding from a private foundation, County Tipperary in Ireland has developed a 'Five Steps to Living Well with Dementia' programme that provides support for people with dementia from the pre-diagnosis to end of life stages, including offering help from Dementia Support Workers and 'community connectors' who can help people with dementia connect with resources and services in the area. Outside of County Tipperary, there are four case managers across Ireland – three operating in the public system, including one supporting elderly patients more generally, and one employed by the Alzheimer's Association. Where case management services are unavailable, primary care physicians often refer people with dementia to public health nurses, who can undertake a care needs assessment, or the Alzheimer's Society of Ireland, for further support.

Online resources are also frequently available for people with dementia and their families to consult. PREPARE, a project to train primary care physicians in dementia management driven by a primary care practitioner in County Cork, Ireland, has developed a website with information on organisations providing support to people with dementia in the country. Alzheimer's Associations are active on a local level in nearly all OECD countries, and frequently have websites that direct people with dementia to locally available resources. Nevertheless, online resources are unlikely to replace support from individuals familiar with the complexities of accessing and qualifying for health and social care services. The advanced age of many people with dementia (and often their carers) may further hinder their access to web-based resources.

Many countries have developed generalised care co-ordination services that serve people with many conditions, including dementia

Across the OECD, a number of countries have facilitated access to care co-ordination and case management through established, generalised pathways of care that were not developed specifically for dementia. In many of these cases, the systems have been developed with enough flexibility to meet the needs of people with dementia. In Norway, municipalities are responsible for care co-ordination and are required to have a coordinating unit available to provide co-ordination services to all residents who require services from more than one agency. Coordinating units offer general co-ordination services and are neither dementia specific nor trained to care for people with dementia. However, municipalities are given flexibility in identifying the most appropriate co-ordinators for each case. Municipality-led dementia memory teams can complement this general care co-ordination and provide pre- and post-diagnostic support for people with dementia. The coordinator identified by the coordinating unit often comes from the memory team, facilitating both continuity in support and allowing for the person with dementia to receive co-ordination services offered by someone familiar with dementia and the resources available to support living with it.

Generalised case management services also operate in Sweden, where all residents have the right to a case manager when needed. Case management is not dementia specific, and many case managers are not trained in dementia care specifically, though training programmes are increasingly available. In Estonia, case management is the responsibility of the municipality, with social workers supporting case management across conditions and diseases, based on need. In Austria, each of the nine Bundesländer has one care organisation responsible for providing case management and care services.

While these case management services can connect people with dementia across the health and social care services they need, most case management programmes are only accessible to people who have met certain thresholds of eligibility. In New Zealand and Canada, for example, level of need is measured using the interRAI assessment system, while in Austria, people in need of care services are assigned to one of seven levels of care support. Though the rationale for a needs-based case management system is clear, in cases where post-diagnostic services are otherwise poorly coordinated, such general case management systems run the risk of excluding some people with dementia who may not yet be in need of home care services, but who should still be connected with the resources available to support them in understanding their diagnosis and the life changes that come with it. In Austria, the need for post-diagnostic support above and beyond existing case management systems has been recognised, with pilot projects underway in Vienna and the region of Tyrol to provide case management services to people with dementia who live at home.

Table 3.1. Availability of care co-ordination services in selected OECD countries

Country	General case management available	General dementia CM	Dementia CM for specific populations
Australia	x		x
Austria	x	Pilot and local initiatives only	
Belgium	x		
Chile	x	Local programmes only	
Czech Republic			
Denmark	x	x	x
Estonia	x		x
Finland	x	x	
France			x
Germany	x		
Greece			
Hungary			
Ireland	x		
Mexico			
Netherlands	x	x	x
Norway	x	x	x
New Zealand	x		
Portugal	x	x	
Slovakia			
Slovenia			
Sweden	x		
Switzerland	x		
United Kingdom (England)		x	
United States	x	Local programmes and pilot initiatives	

Source: OECD Dementia Survey and Interviews 2016-2017.

In some health systems, post-diagnostic care pathways have been designed specifically for people with dementia

Formalised, dementia-specific care pathways including case management components have in some cases been developed to help people navigate health and social care following a dementia diagnosis. Using existing case management pathways can in many cases allows people living with dementia to be connected with case managers and other professionals who are intimately familiar with the array of health and social care services available in the area. But for people with dementia whose needs may not yet meet the care thresholds required to access existing case management support, the information they receive following diagnosis may be determined more by what their clinician is familiar with than what might actually be available. For these cases, dementia-specific care pathways can help people to get the services they need. In Denmark, each of the five administrative regions is responsible for developing care pathways for people living with dementia. In the Capital region of Denmark, hospitals, primary care clinics, memory clinics, and municipalities – which are responsible for rehabilitation, preventive services, social care, and home care – work together to coordinate responsibilities with relation to people with dementia. In most cases of dementia, a nurse employed by the municipality is responsible for organising home care services, while the patient's general practitioner will act as their medical coordinator and be responsible for all health-related services. General practitioners are required to follow up with their patients with dementia at least once per year. For the annual dementia visits, general practitioners receive an additional fee of about EUR 100. For complex cases, home care is managed by a specialised nurse coordinator at a memory clinic, while a specialist from the same memory clinic is responsible for clinical co-ordination.

In Norway, municipal memory teams provide both pre- and post-diagnostic support to people diagnosed with dementia. The memory teams are distinct from Norway's more general care co-ordination, which is available to any individuals requiring services from more than one health or social care agency. Norway's national guidelines recommend all people with dementia receive support from a coordinator, even before they qualify for existing co-ordination services. Often the first point of contact where someone is concerned about possible cognitive troubles, memory teams also follow up in the aftermath of a dementia diagnosis. It is recommended that people with dementia are reassessed by memory teams after six months, including whether they need services such as day care placement or support for caregiving relatives.

A similar model of care is available in Scotland and some parts of Australia, where the position of a 'dementia link worker' has been established to help people with dementia and their families access the support services they need. The government of Scotland requires that all people diagnosed with dementia as of April 2013 receive a minimum of one year of post-diagnostic support (Alzheimer's Scotland, 2017). Achievement of this target is monitored through the inclusion indicators monitoring new dementia diagnoses and linkage to support workers through the Local Delivery Plan NHS performance standards (NHS National Services Scotland, 2017).

Offering both dementia-specific and more general support is similarly the model in Japan, where case management is an integral part of national goals to support elderly citizens to age in the community, through the Integrated Community Care System (Ministry of Health, Labour and Welfare, 2017). The country's 'Orange Plan' dementia strategy further calls for the development of dementia care pathways to be implemented at the municipal level throughout Japan. In addition to services offered through integrated community support centres. Japan recently developed integrated care teams for early dementia. Teams are located in integrated community support centres, but also offer home visits, assessments, and support to family members of people with early onset dementia.

In the United States, a number of locally-based case management programmes have been demonstrated to improve health outcomes and reduce costs in dementia care. In Los Angeles, California, the University of California at Los Angeles (UCLA) has developed an Alzheimer's and Dementia Care programme, in which all patients receive support from a geriatric nurse practitioner assigned to act as their case manager. The programme is aimed at improving care and health outcomes while reducing healthcare costs and use of healthcare services. It aims to do so by targeting three perceived gaps in care: 1) improving support and training for caregivers; 2) improving transitions in care settings; and 3) improving access to community-based services (Tan, Jennings and Reuben, 2014, Reuben et al., 2013). Similar case management programmes have been adopted by hospital systems in other parts of the United States, including San Diego, California, and Indiana (Reuben et al., 2013).

Case management can help to identify and coordinate needed services for people with dementia

Reviews of case management programmes for people with dementia suggest that in at least some cases, case management can improve quality of life for people with dementia and their carers, help delay transitions to care, and increase service utilisation (Vickrey et al., 2006, Parker et al., 2008). However, existing evidence suggests that case management does not necessarily deliver these benefits under all circumstances. While further evidence around the impact of case management on people living with dementia is needed, a number of general conclusions that impact the way co-ordination is delivered can be drawn.

Many countries have established formalised case management programmes open to people with dementia and other conditions. These programmes are most often based on a minimum level of assessed need, or open to people who require services from two or more separate agencies. In many cases, people newly diagnosed with dementia may not yet meet the criteria necessary to receive case management services. It has been suggested that earlier case management interventions may lead to greater satisfaction with the service among informal carers (Peeters et al., 2016). Given the importance of ensuring caregiver quality of life and support in caring, better satisfaction with case management services could possibly translate into lower burden among carers and better outcomes for people with dementia.

However, other studies comparing case management to regular post-diagnostic care among people with early stages of dementia have found no difference in effect on quality of life, caregiver burden, or depressive symptoms among people living with dementia or their carers (Jansen et al., 2011). It is possible that the length of follow-up in most studies may not adequately capture the longer-term effects of earlier interventions. Studies with longer follow-up times appear to more strongly demonstrate a delayed effect on institutionalisation from case management (Koch et al., 2012). Implementing case management interventions at earlier stages of dementia may also be more effective in settings where 'normal' care is less comprehensive and people with dementia and their carers receive less information from their primary care physicians on accessing relevant health and social care services.

There is substantial evidence to suggest that intensive models of case management may deliver higher-quality case management for people with dementia and their family carers. Intensive care management, in which the case manager and care agencies operate within one network, have been suggested to improve quality of life to a greater degree than linked care models, where case managers connect people with dementia to multiple competing agencies (van Mierlo et al., 2014; Vroomen et al., 2015).

A randomised control trial of different models of case management in the Netherlands suggests that intensive care co-ordination is likely needed for case management to be successful, but that the higher costs associated with intensive co-ordination may detract from any cost effectiveness delivered by the intervention (van Mierlo et al., 2004; Vroomen et al., 2012; Khanassov, Vedel and Pluye, 2014).

Targeted care co-ordination or case management for people with complex needs can be effective

Very often, people living with dementia also have one or more co-morbidities that make supporting their long-term health and care needs much more complex. In these cases, people may require services from an array of health and social care organisations, and the level or intensity of support may change over time. Navigating through the organisational complexity of accessing care and support from different points in the health and social system can be overwhelming, even without the cognitive problems people with dementia face. People facing early onset dementia or those from minority cultural or language backgrounds can also face additional difficulties accessing relevant services, particularly where they are designed for more 'typical' patients. In these cases, offering personalised support to people living with dementia, and their families, can help ensure that they receive the services they need.

In France, the *Maisons pour l'Autonomie et l'Intégration des Malades Alzheimer* (MAIA) provide a single point of entry to health and long-term care services for people with very complex cases of dementia. MAIA is a form of integrated care management that helps people with high needs access the services they need across health and social care settings. While the definition of "complex" cases differs by MAIA, most people will have behavioural needs or major health issues and face difficulty receiving care from informal carers or other existing caregivers. The programme helps to facilitate co-ordination between stakeholders providing health, social and administrative services related to dementia care, including health insurance, health services, retirement insurance, and social security through strategic consultation and the appointment of a "local pilot" tasked with coordinating relevant stakeholders (Pimouguet, 2013). Relevant services are then made available to people with dementia through an integrated service window that provides one entry point to accessing a range of services including health care-related needs and access to hospitals, hospital at home services, housing services, and mobile geriatric care services. People with dementia then receive personalised case management, including individual care plans, to ensure that their needs are met. Based on the PRISMA model of care co-ordination in Quebec, Canada, MAIA were developed as part of the 2008-2012 French National Alzheimer Plan (Pimouguet, 2013). More than 350 MAIA had been developed throughout France by the end of 2016. Not all people with dementia qualify for case management and support through MAIA. More recently, the MAIA model was expanded to include others with complex needs who do not have dementia.

In Estonia, people with early onset dementia are eligible for a separate system of support, provided through the National Insurance Board. Qualifying patients receive state care services, including individual case management services and personalised rehabilitation plans. While the programme is not limited to those with dementia (among others, people with schizophrenia and other psychiatric conditions are also eligible), special care services only support people with dementia under the age of 65, after which they must use the services available in their local municipality. Special case management programmes for people with early onset dementia are similarly available in Australia, where the National Younger Onset Dementia Key Worker Program, funded by the Department of Social Services, provides case management support to people under the age of 65. People with symptoms of dementia who have not yet been diagnosed are also eligible for support through the Dementia Key Worker Program, in the event of which case managers can help people to obtain a formal diagnosis.

Improving the co-ordination of care is critical to ensure people with dementia have timely access to the services they need. OECD countries have adopted a range of approaches to improving care co-ordination, and should continue to focus on improving post-diagnostic care and support for people with dementia. Countries that have not developed care co-ordination or case management pathways for people with dementia should consider whether such programmes would help to improve service co-ordination, particularly for people with complex needs.

Some countries have created community-based dementia staff positions to help people with dementia and their families better navigate life in the community

As ageing in the community becomes more common, communities have begun to develop new professional staff positions and resource centres focused on supporting people with dementia who live in the community. These positions are sometimes located in existing health or social services, and frequently focus their support exclusively on people with dementia or other cognitive difficulties. They can provide services similar to case managers or care co-ordinators, and are often the first point of contact for people with dementia or their carers, even before a formal diagnosis has been made.

Community-based memory "teams" or dementia coordinator positions can help people with dementia and their families to prepare for a possible dementia diagnosis, understand and process its implications, and connect them with available resources. In Norway, so-called 'memory teams' operate in 75% of municipalities across the country. Made up of health professionals, occupational therapists, and other health and social staff trained in dementia care, memory teams can be contacted by people with dementia or their families even before a diagnosis has been made and are equipped to perform comprehensive initial diagnostic assessments, including during home visits. Memory teams further provide follow-up support after a diagnosis for at least six months. Members of the memory team are often appointed the official care coordinator for people living with dementia, allowing for further continuity in care. In Denmark, most municipalities have dementia co-ordinators who perform similar functions, visiting people concerned about dementia symptoms prior to a diagnostic evaluation, and offering help in coordinating care after a diagnosis is made. A network of memory nurses across Finland, located in primary healthcare clinics, perform similar counselling and coordinating functions for people with dementia and their families, particularly those with advanced forms of the disease who live in the community.

Chile has adopted a community-based approach to dementia care with the development of a new "community manager" role. Based on the recognition that the gap between dementia prevalence and diagnosis is very high in Chile, the government has introduced this position to help identify, on the very local level, people who may have dementia who have not yet accessed the health system and received a diagnostic evaluation. Community managers use their knowledge of the local community to perform an active case-finding role. Community managers also follow up with people who are known to have dementia and live in the community, performing home visits and other follow-up to ensure they receive the care they need. Unlike memory teams and dementia co-ordinators, who are trained in dementia care and often come from the health or social care sectors, community managers are not expected to be health or care professionals, but are instead often themselves older, sometimes retired adults who are re-employed for their new position. This approach offers an interesting model in integrating dementia care at the very local community level. The older age profile of community managers, and their semi-professional background, may also be advantageous connecting with people socially, and in reassuring those who might be less comfortable receiving visits or care from formal health and social services.

3.3. Making communities work for people with dementia

3.3.1. Dementia-friendly communities can improve quality of life in the community for people with dementia

Even as countries have increasingly focused on encouraging community-based living for older populations, people with dementia frequently face challenges that make staying in the community particularly difficult. These include problems related to unintentional wandering, challenges with driving and using public transportation, difficulties in the home environment, a lack of understanding from people in the community, including in the service industry, and exploitation, such as elder abuse and fraud. Designing interventions that can help to reduce the risks people with dementia living in the community face is critical to allowing people to age in place while maintaining a high quality of life. These policies address not only the broader community, but must also target the quality of life of informal carers.

Box 3.1. Care in the community

People living with dementia can live for a long period or even their entire life at home, if they receive adequate support and long-term care. Long-term care can be delivered through formal services, but also through family members or friends (Colombo, F. et al., 2011). People with dementia can receive long-term care both at home or in long-term care facilities. In this report, we refer to community-based care as services and support that is offered to people with dementia that enables them to live at home, whether or not they receive (formal or informal) long-term care services.

Over the past decade, interventions focused on promoting dementia-friendliness have been increasingly adopted in countries around the world to allow people living with dementia to feel included and supported in their communities (Heward et al., 2017). The concept of dementia-friendly communities initially emerged in Japan, where serious efforts have been undertaken to destigmatise dementia and sensitise communities to be more accepting and inclusive of people living with the disease (Aihara et al., 2016). Dementia-friendly communities aim to help people living with dementia to stay in their communities longer. But beyond more pragmatic goals of making communities easier to live in for people with dementia, they also aim to promote acceptance of people with dementia as active and important members of their communities, reduce stigma and improve understanding of dementia.

Programmes that tackle behaviours like wandering can make communities easier to navigate for people living with dementia

Some OECD communities have developed programmes that address specific behaviours or characteristics exhibited by people with dementia which can put them at risk. Wandering behaviour, for example, is linked with higher risk of injury – including an increased risk of falls – and higher carer stress (Douglas et al., 2011; Logsdon et al., 1998). Wandering is a major concern for individuals living with dementia in community settings; a substantial proportion of people with dementia living in the community exhibit wandering behaviour, with some estimates suggesting that as many as four in five people with dementia in the community wander at some point (Klein et al., 1999; Hope et al., 1994; Hope et al., 2001). In Japan, the SOS Wanderers Network was established as a neighbourhood watch-style network to engage the community to search for people with dementia who may have wandered away and are missing (Hayashi, 2016). Local police alert members of the wanderer's network – consisting of community residents, local business, and local media – when a person with dementia goes missing. In 2014, over 10 000 people were reported missing to the wanderer's network (Hayashi, 2016). The programme, which started in the municipality of Omuta in 2001, has since scaled nationally, with 40% of Local Authorities establishing similar models (Hayashi, 2016).

Box 3.2. What's in a name? Strategies to reduce stigma and increase awareness for dementia in Japan

As one of the most rapidly ageing countries in the world, Japan has faced the challenges of an increasingly ageing population more quickly than many other OECD countries. The share of the population aged over 65, and over 85, is the highest in the OECD, at 27% and 8%, respectively (OECD, 2017). By 2050, current estimates indicate that 36% of the population will be older than 65, and 15% will be over 85. To prepare for its ageing population, Japan has introduced significant reforms to its long-term care system in the past decades, most notably through the introduction of the Long-Term Care Insurance (LTCI) programme in 2000. Compared with most other OECD countries, the proportion of the elderly population receiving care at home is high: as one measure, the number of long-term care beds in institutions and hospitals in 2015 was the fifth-lowest in the OECD (OECD, 2017). Japan's social care system reflects this, with a strong emphasis on providing community-based comprehensive care for the elderly (Hayashi, 2015).

In recent years, the country has taken important steps toward making its communities more liveable for people with dementia and their families. As a part of a move to reduce the stigma associated with the disease, the official name for dementia was changed in 2004. The process, which included public consultation, aimed to develop an alternative name for dementia that conveyed the seriousness of the condition but did not carry the strong stigma attached to the previous name (Miyamoto et al., 2011). A similar re-naming was previously undertaken for other cognitive disorders, including schizophrenia. Research indicates that the change in name and accompanying awareness campaigns helped to reduce the stigma around schizophrenia. Similarly, there is evidence that people with dementia have begun to increasingly speak in public about the condition since the change in name (Koike et al., 2015). Similar approaches to renaming dementia have been considered in other Asian countries where the name for dementia has insulting or stigmatising connotations (Chiu et al., 2014).

Alongside the official name change for dementia, from chiho to ninchisho, the government launched an ambitious public campaign that aimed to build awareness and understanding around dementia (Miyamoto et al., 2011). The 10-Year Plan to Understand Dementia and Build Community Networks comprised four components, including training one million dementia supporters, developing dementia-friendly communities, creating support groups for people with dementia and their families, and providing case management for people with dementia and their carers.

Japan's experience integrating its launch of a new name for dementia with an ambitious community-based sensitisation programme offers an interesting lesson in how messaging can be creatively used to re-sensitise communities to a previously highly stigmatised disease like dementia. It is possible that people were more receptive to the awareness campaigns given the new name and positive way in which they were conducted.

In the United States, a number of states have adopted an alert system to solicit community support when a person with dementia goes missing. Modelled after the alert system adopted for child abductions, Silver Alerts disseminate missing-persons alerts across social media, local media outlets and roadway signs to alert the public. Thirty six US states currently use Silver Alert programmes to engage the community in helping find people with dementia who are missing.

Engaging local businesses, public services, and community members can improve the daily life of people with dementia

Over 90% of OECD countries have in place at least some dementia-friendly activities. In addition to developing community interventions that address specific behaviours exhibited by people with dementia, some communities have developed dementia-friendly awareness and training programmes specifically for certain public and private sectors that are likely to come into contact with people with dementia. However, in almost all cases, such activities are organised on an ad-hoc or voluntary basis, and their availability can vary significantly even within one country.

In Austria, an interactive training programme for police officers has been implemented through the Security Academy of the Interior Ministry. The internet-based training, taught in three short modules, helps police officers to recognise a person who may have dementia and teaches them behavioural strategies to help de-escalate situations in which people with dementia may be agitated or otherwise exhibiting behavioural or psychological symptoms of dementia. Police stations with high participation can apply to have their station certified as dementia-friendly. 70% of police officers in the police station must have completed at least one module and passed an exam related to the training. The station must further demonstrate that they engage with the broader community in dementia awareness, such as working with staff at nursing homes to address wandering and other behavioural challenges. Since the programme was established in 2013, 25 police stations have been certified, with 2 000 police officers trained in dementia awareness and response.

A number of countries have developed programmes to improve dementia awareness among pharmacists. Given their role in distributing medicine and frequent contact with patients, pharmacists have a unique role to play in helping people with dementia, particularly with regard to taking steps to ensure they continue to take any needed medications and observing changes in their behaviour over time. Pharmacists often have long-term, trusting relationships with their patients and often have a comprehensive view of the multiple conditions many of their patients with dementia may be living with (Pharmaceutical Society of Australia, 2014). In Flanders, Belgium, the Flemish Pharmacist Network has worked with the Flemish Dementia Expertise Centre to increase the role of pharmacists, together with primary care practitioners, in supporting people with dementia. The programme, which was rolled out in February 2017, aims to train pharmacists throughout Flanders to ensure they have the necessary knowledge and information to both identify the first signs of dementia and provide information and support, including referrals on to further services, to people living with dementia and their family members. Similar dementia-friendly pharmacy initiatives have been developed in other OECD countries, including Australia, Canada, the United Kingdom, and the United States.

Most dementia-friendly training programmes targeting the general public require relatively low financial and time investments. Becoming a dementia friend in the United Kingdom, for example, requires attending a one-hour information session, or registering online and viewing an informational video. Where engaged, private companies have proven receptive to supporting efforts to increase awareness about dementia. In the United Kingdom, large businesses including Marks and Spencer's, Lloyd's Bank, and Superdrug have trained their staff to become dementia friends. By 2014, the enrolment of dementia friends through the business sector was twice that of targets set by the Prime Minister's Challenge (Donnelly, 2014). By 2020, the country aims to have 25% of FTSE 500 companies certified as dementia friendly. Dementia friendly charters have been developed separately for the financial services, technology, housing, and retail sectors. In encouraging large businesses to become involved in dementia friendly initiatives, countries can expand the reach of their campaigns at relatively low cost. Companies also benefit, with their involvement helping to reflect an image of corporate social responsibility and commitment to social inclusion, two values increasingly important in the corporate environment. Dementia-friendly initiatives have frequently been spearheaded by non-governmental organisations and advocacy groups. In Germany, for example, Aktion Demenz has played an important role in promoting dementia-friendly communities across the country.

Box 3.3. Promoting dementia-friendly communities in England

Ensuring communities are able to help people living with dementia live independently was a major focus of the Prime Minister's 2020 Challenge on Dementia. As part of this challenge, the Alzheimer's Society, with support from the Department of Health, developed foundation criteria for recognising dementia-friendly communities across England. Support for dementia-friendly initiatives far exceeded initial targets. By March 2015, 98 communities had met the foundation criteria, surpassing the initial goal of reaching 20 communities by 2015. Today, more than 192 communities have been registered in the dementia-friendly foundation process – an area that covers a population of more than 26 million people. To provide clearer guidelines to communities interested in qualifying as dementia-friendly, in 2015, a Publically Available Specification for dementia friendly communities was developed in concert with the Department of Health and British Standards Institute.

3.3.2. Measuring outcomes for people with dementia living in the community

There is little standardised measurement of outcomes for people living with dementia in the community

At present, few countries evaluate how people with dementia live in the community in a regular or comprehensive manner. Eight of 21 OECD countries (38%) reported that they could estimate the proportion of people with dementia who live in the community, though they do not always do so. Eleven out of 21 OECD countries (52%) can identify people who have received a diagnosis of dementia and receive long-term care services at home. In Australia, the number of claims made for the Dementia and Cognition Supplement for home care packages can be used as a proxy for the number of people with dementia who live at home, though not all people with dementia require home care packages and not all who could benefit necessarily apply for the supplement. In Finland, a diagnosis of dementia is included in the social care registry that tracks both facility-based and home care services, and can serve as a similar proxy tool. Using the dementia registry SveDem and other tools, information on living conditions and treatment and care data, including prescriptions data and information about access to day care services, can be combined for people with dementia in Sweden. This kind of detailed information allows researchers and policymakers to determine whether people with dementia living at home are receiving the support they need.

Table 3.2. Data availability for community-based measures for people with dementia

	Proportion of people with dementia who live in the community	People with a dementia diagnosis who receive LTC at home
Australia	National data Can be estimated through a combination of survey and residential aged care sources. Not previously attempted.	National data Claims numbers for the Dementia and Cognition Supplement
Austria		Local or regional data
Canada	National data	National data Home Care Reporting System (HCRS) - clinical and administrative data collected for long-stay home care clients using the RAI Home Care assessment. Coverage includes seven provinces/territories four of which have complete coverage). Database also includes additional data from Ontario using the interRAI-Contact Assessment which is used to make decisions about home care eligibility.
Czech Republic		
Denmark		
Finland	National data	National data Social care register includes people with a dementia diagnosis who live at home and receive home care services
France	National data	Local/regional data
Ireland		National data Population-level survey data from The Irish Longitudinal Study on Aging (TILDA) (uses a representative sample of 8,000 adults aged 50 and older)
Israel	Local/regional data Health maintenance organisations record information on community health care in medical records	National data Since 2014, data available through National Insurance Institute database on long-term care at home.
Japan		National data
Latvia		
Luxembourg		National data
Mexico	National data	
Netherlands		
Norway	National data IPLOS registry records information on municipal health and care services	National data
Poland		National data
Slovakia		Local/regional data
Spain		
Sweden	National data Matching several data sources (SveDem, BPSD, SPDR, National Patient Register, Register for Social Service for Disabled and Elderly	National data
Switzerland		National data
United Kingdom (Northern Ireland)		
United Kingdom (Scotland)	National data	National data Administrative data from care at home providers
United Kingdom (Wales)		
Total countries with national data (/23)	**8**	**12**

Source: 2016-17 OECD Dementia Survey and Interviews.

Because there is no cure for dementia, many of the interventions in place to help people with the condition are focused as much if not more on improving well-being and quality of life as improving cognition. Yet measures of quality of life – including person- and carer-reported measures – are notably absent from regular data collections and measurement in nearly all OECD countries. Just two countries – Australia and Canada, reported that they have tools to regularly measure wellbeing or quality of life of people with dementia on a national level. In Australia, quality of life measures for people with dementia have come from national surveys, including the National Health Survey and Survey of Disability, Ageing and Carers, a regularly repeated national survey that includes questions related to function and community participation. Information about clinical outcomes (such as pain), functional ability, and social participation (such as visits) for people with dementia is available in Canada through the Continuing Care Reporting System and the Home Care Reporting System. In Denmark, the national dementia registry, launched in 2016, will collect person-reported indicators. Increasing the use of person-reported indicators is also under consideration in the SveDem registry in Sweden. An evaluation of eight European countries – Estonia, Finland, France, Germany, the Netherlands, Spain, Sweden, and the United Kingdom (England) – examined how quality of life and quality of care differed across where people with dementia lived (care facilities versus at home), and found significant variation between countries, though not between settings (Beerens et al., 2014). Quality of life for people with dementia living in the community has been measured more extensively as part of research on specific interventions or academic studies.

In addition to generic tools developed to evaluate person-reported measures, such as the EQ5D, quality of life for people with dementia living in the community has been measured more extensively as part of research on specific interventions or academic studies (Algar et al., 2016). Many tools exist to measure person-reported outcomes in the dementia population. A recent review identified fifteen separate instruments to measure health-related quality of life in people with Alzheimer's disease and other dementias (Perales et al., 2013). However, person-report outcome and experience measures have been less frequently used outside the research context for people with dementia, and are not well integrated into regular data collection mechanisms in most OECD countries. In the United Kingdom (England and Scotland), four health economies have begun piloting a standard set of dementia outcome measures developed by the International Consortium of Health Outcomes Measurement (ICHOM). ICHOM's standard set, which was developed with the input of experts, people with dementia and their carers, includes indicators that use person- and carer-reported measures to evaluate quality of life. Memory assessment services, liaison services (to care homes and acute hospitals), mental health ward services, and community teams (who make home visits) are involved in collecting the standard set. In Doncaster – one of the three English sites for the pilot – data collected through the dementia standard set is being used to inform post-diagnostic service commissioning.

Box 3.4. The ICHOM Dementia Implementation Community

The International Consortium for Health Outcomes Measurement (ICHOM) is a non-profit organisation focused on promoting value-based health care through the definition and dissemination of disease-specific outcome measures that emphasises what matters to patients. As part of this work, ICHOM – in partnership with people with dementia, their carers, researchers, and clinicians, developed a Dementia Standard Set for people living with dementia.

In July 2016, a 'Dementia Implementation Community' was formed, involving three 'health economies' across NHS England to assess the feasibility of the ICHOM Dementia Standard Set, across health and social care. Organisations across Central and North West (CNW) London, Doncaster and Manchester, collectively implemented the set with the support of ICHOM. Through community teleconferences, health economies shared their learnings and collectively work together to achieve key milestones in the process and define the opportunities as well as logistical challenges of implementation.

Each health economy, having reviewed their commissioned dementia services, resources and current practice in data collection, selected to implement different indicators across different services within the care pathway. The selected indicators reflected clinical interest to further understand and evaluate the quality of service provision and its effect on patient outcomes.

A key objective of the pilot was to define the feasibility of implementing the set in clinical settings. In Doncaster, for example, an initial output highlighted the appropriateness of implementing questionnaires, such as the MoCA, amongst patients with varying levels of disease severity. A second objective was to evaluate the use of data to assess service provision. Pilot data collected in Doncaster is currently being used to inform the commissioning of services and staff, particularly in post-diagnostic support services.

Furthermore, the pilot has highlighted the importance of deploying a scalable data collection platform, particularly one that enables access to data across specialties and services involved in patient care. Following the initial phase of the pilot, the next step is to continue to pilot the patient-reported outcome measure questionnaires and variables in the set and reevaluate their use in additional settings. In Manchester, for example, the initial data collected will be reviewed alongside the results of a clinical trial and the pilot extended to a specialized clinic setting. The collation and analysis of data commenced in September 2017 with a report to follow. The team in central and northwest London is continuing data collection across their selected sites and intend to design an organisation-wide quality improvement and evaluation process, whereby outcomes data is used to evaluate the impact of applied change initiatives.

Defining and measuring the impact of dementia-friendly community policies remains a challenge

Dementia-friendly initiatives have been promoted and advanced in nearly all national dementia strategies or plans in OECD countries. Building a dementia-friendly society is frequently cited as the overarching goal of the national policy document. But what this means in practice is often less clear, with few countries supplying clear outcome goals for measuring what is meant by dementia friendliness, and when it can be considered to have been achieved.

In the United Kingdom (England), measures of dementia-friendliness have been clearly incorporated into the Prime Minister's Challenge on Dementia 2020. An implementation plan developed together with the Challenge outlines targets for achieving dementia friendly communities, including making 50% of all Local Authority areas (a total of 75 Local Authorities) and 25% of FTSE 500 companies dementia-friendly by 2020 (Challenge on Dementia 2020 Implementation Plan, 2016). These targets build on ambitious goals set during the first Prime Minister's Challenge on Dementia, launched in 2012, which aimed to train one million people to become "dementia friends" and helped to launch awareness about building dementia-friendly communities in the United Kingdom. Similar programmes were developed in the early 2000s in Japan, which in 2005 launched a "10-Year Plan to Understand Dementia and Build Community Networks." Launched amid a national drive to reduce stigma and increase awareness for dementia which included an official renaming of dementia in Japanese, the campaign also aimed to train one million "dementia supporters" through a three-level training approach. Both countries exceeded initial goals for training dementia friends: As of June 2017, more than two million people had been trained as dementia friends in the United Kingdom, while in Japan, 9.5 million people (as of June 2017) had attended training seminars by September 2014, with nearly all municipalities in the country offering training programmes by 2015 (Alzheimer's Disease International, 2017).

Japan and the United Kingdom (England) represent two uncommon examples of countries that have developed explicit targets to measure progress towards achieving dementia-friendly communities. Even in these countries, however, the chosen indicators can be seen to be 'intermediate' measures that count outputs – such as dementia friends, or the number of dementia-friendly communities – rather than outcomes, such as improvements in quality of life or delayed time to institutionalisation among people with dementia. Given the range of activities that can be considered "dementia-friendly," and the difficulty of isolating community interventions from other influencing factors, it is challenging to link the impact of dementia friendly interventions with outcome measures such as health outcomes or even delays in institutionalisation. As dementia-friendly programmes become more commonplace, there has been some increase in research on the subject. In England, the Department of Health recently commissioned a research study, led by the University of Hertfordshire, to evaluate the evidence base for dementia-friendly communities. Patient- and carer-reported measures may offer an opportunity to develop an understanding of the impact of these programmes on the quality of life of people with dementia and their families.

3.4. Better support for families and informal carers

3.4.1. Supporting informal carers is a crucial part of dementia care

OECD countries increasingly promote community-based care and ageing in place, and the role played by informal carers will become even more important. It may also be more challenging. As people stay in the community with increasingly advanced cases of dementia which would previously have been cared for in institutional or inpatient settings, carers may be tasked with providing with more intensive or complex care. The burden of providing informal care, particularly for people with dementia, affects the physical and mental health and quality of life of the carer. It can also influence the health of those they care for. Informal carers play an integral role in caring for people with dementia. It is crucial that policies that work to improve the quality of life and health outcomes of people with dementia must also consider those who care for them.

What constitutes informal care can be challenging to define and difficult to compare. Informal carers may provide care to friends or family members, or may do so as part of non-contractual voluntary work. They may also be undeclared or illegal caregivers who receive a salary or compensation from the care recipient, but do not have an official contract with them and are not registered with relevant social security offices. In the following section, we focus our attention on informal caregivers who are family members, friends, or uncompensated volunteers who provide support to care recipients on a regular basis and who do not receive cash or other benefits beyond those intended to support caring activities.

Many people living with dementia rely on their families and other informal carers

Across the OECD, more than one in eight adults over fifty provides informal care to a friend or family member (with or without dementia) at least once per week (Figure 3.2). The variation in informal caring varies substantially between countries, ranging from 8% in Poland to more than 20% in the Czech Republic. The intensity of caring also varies: though more than 10% of adults over 50 in the Czech Republic provide informal caring services on a daily basis, just 4% do so in Switzerland and Sweden. Lower rates of more intensive (daily) caregiving are seen in countries where the formal long-term care sector is better developed. Even before the challenges that can come with caring for friends of family members living with dementia, older adults regularly face their own health challenges.

Informal carers appear to carry a higher burden of care for people with dementia in countries with less developed or comprehensive long-term care sectors. In an evaluation of the economic impact of dementia in Europe, the costs of informal care were estimated to represent 40% of the total costs of dementia in Northern and Western Europe, but 75% of the total costs of dementia in Southern and Eastern Europe (Wimo et al., 2011). Informal care costs can include the cost of unpaid labour provided by informal carers, the opportunity costs associated with forgoing work in order to provide care, and the direct out-of-pocket costs that informal carers spend on care. A recent analysis of the economic costs of dementia in Chile similarly found that 75% of total dementia costs could be attributed to informal care and other indirect costs and found that even within the country, households of lower socioeconomic status depended more on informal care than households of higher socioeconomic status, who could purchase more formal medical and social care (Hojman et al., 2017).

Figure 3.2. Share of informal carers among population age 50 and over

2015 (or nearest year)

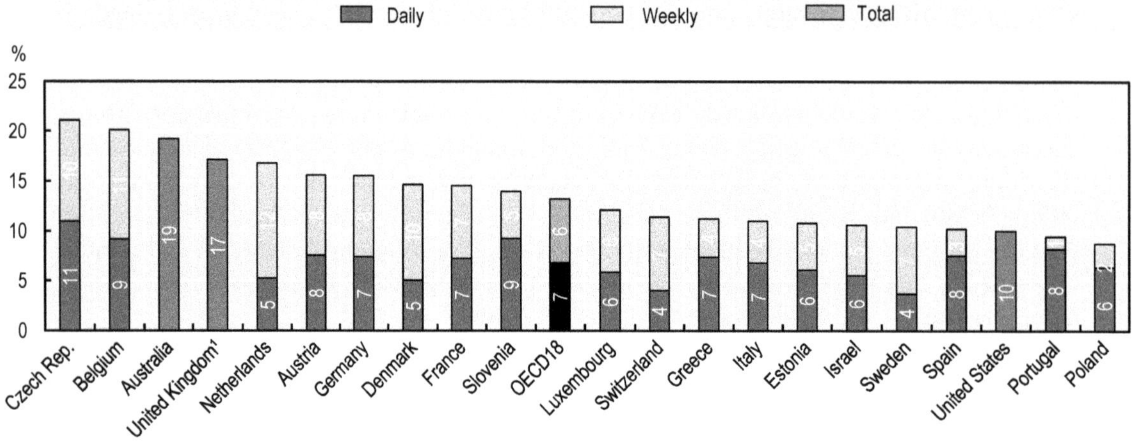

Note: The definition of informal carers differs between surveys. 1. United Kingdom refers to England.
Source: *OECD Health Statistics 2017*, http://dx.doi.org/10.1787/health-data-en.

StatLink http://dx.doi.org/10.1787/888933735234

Figure 3.3. Informal care costs as a share of total dementia costs

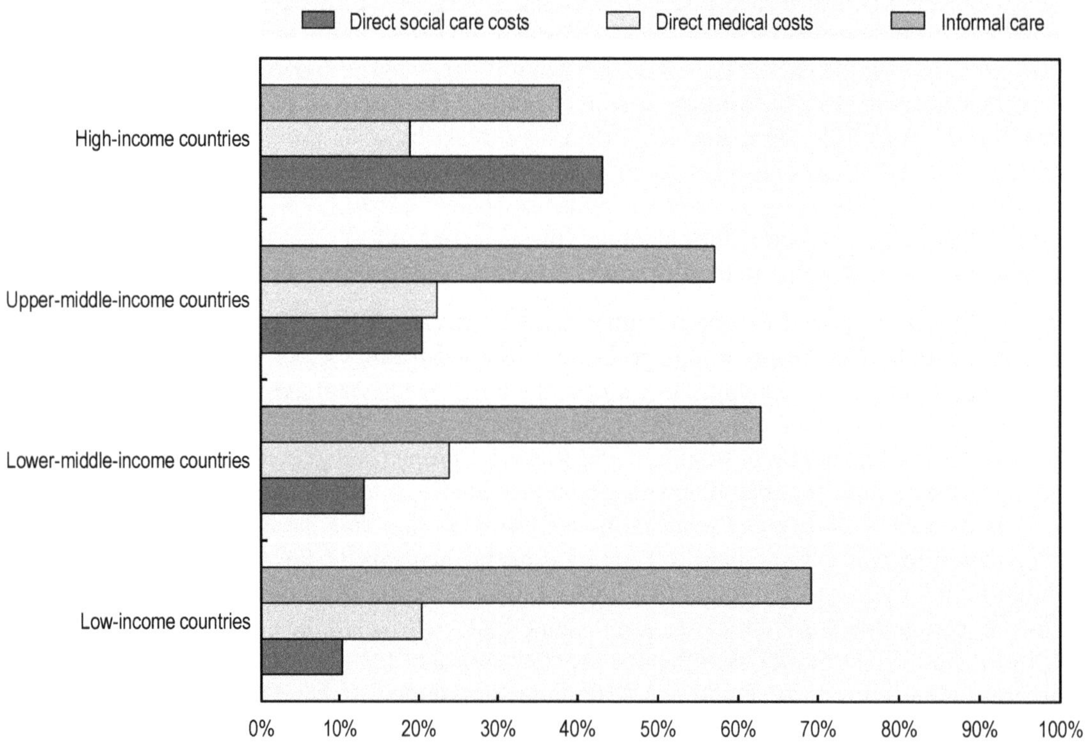

Source: Wimo et al. (2017).

StatLink http://dx.doi.org/10.1787/888933735253

Women make up the majority of informal caregivers in nearly all OECD countries. Across 21 OECD countries, three in five informal carers providing daily care were women (Figure 3.4). Informal carers are less likely to be formally employed, and are more likely to be employed part-time when working, when compared with non-caring workers. Previous analyses have suggested that women carers are particularly at risk of poverty, possibly associated with their lower rates of participation in the labour force (Carmichael and Charles, 2003; Heitmueller, 2007; Viitanen, 2005; Colombo, F. et al., 2011). They may also have been more dependent on their spouse or other friend or family member for whom they are now caring (Colombo, F. et al., 2011).

Figure 3.4. Share of women among informal daily carers aged 50 and over

2015 (or nearest year)

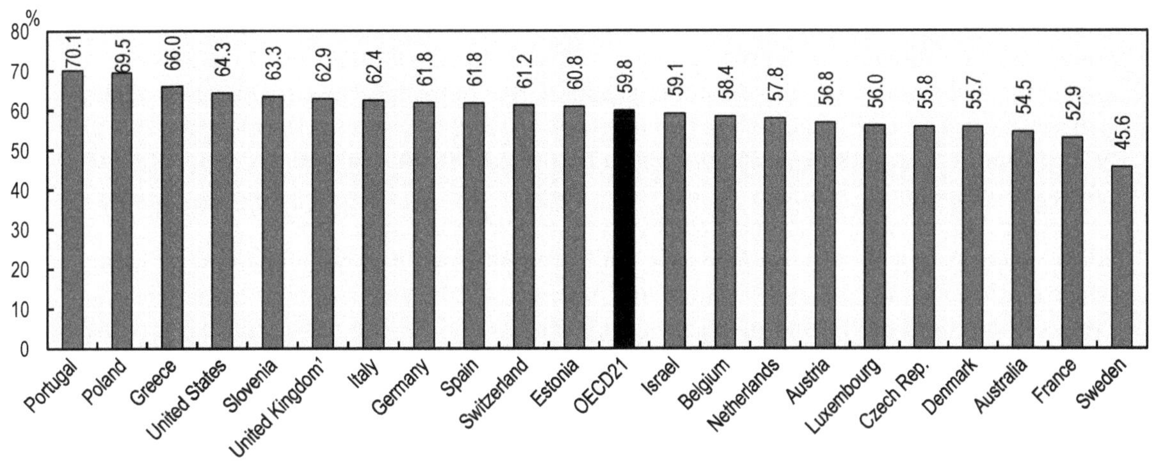

Note: The definition of informal carers differs between surveys. 1. United Kingdom refers to England.
Source: Wave 6 of the Survey of Health, Ageing and Retirement in Europe (2015), Survey of Disability, Ageing and Carers for Australia (2015), wave 7 of the English Longitudinal Study of Ageing (2015), wave 12 of the Health and Retirement Survey for the United States (2014).

StatLink http://dx.doi.org/10.1787/888933735272

Providing informal care is linked with worse health outcomes, particularly mental health

The association between informal caring and poor health outcomes is well documented across studies (Thomas et al., 2015; Stansfeld et al., 2014; Pinquart and Sörensen, 2003; Schulz and Sherwood, 2008; Cannuscio et al., 2002; Ory et al., 1999; Adelman et al., 2014; Chiao, Wu and Hsiao, 2015). A longitudinal study using data from the Nurse's Health Study in the United States found that women who provided intensive caregiving (36 hours or more per week) to a spouse were nearly six times more likely to be depressed or anxious (Cannuscio et al., 2002). Caring for a parent also led to a higher risk of depression and anxiety. Caregivers are much more likely to report poorer subjective quality of life than similar adults who do not care for family or friends (Thomas et al., 2015; Pinquart & Sörensen, 2003). Providing care has also been associated with poorer physical health outcomes, though these effects are smaller than the effects of caring on mental health. People who provide care that includes support for activities of daily living (ADL) have also been found to disregard their own personal well-being, including consuming poorer diets and neglecting to take their own medications or attend doctor's appointments (Schulz and

Sherwood, 2008, Burton et al., 2003). The length and intensity of caring have been associated with higher risks of stress, particularly among women (Hirst, 2005). Given the gradual onset of dementia, many people may find themselves caring for a friend or family member with the disease for an extended period of time, often years.

Caring for people with dementia has been found to negatively affect the health of the caregivers (Etters et al., 2008). Notably, caregivers supporting people living with dementia are much more likely to experience poorer mental and physical health than non-carers and non-dementia caregivers (Pinquart & Sörensen, 2003, Ory et al., 1999). Carers for people with dementia have been found to provide more intensive caring than other carers (Ory et al., 1999). Caregiving burden is particularly high when the person with dementia has high needs, including behavioural and psychological symptoms of dementia (BPSD) (Vaingankar et al., 2016). They report more difficulties with employment, higher overall stress, less time spent on other activities, and more mental and physical health problems than caregivers to people with other conditions (Ory et al., 1999). In Norway, family members were found to spend an average of 160 hours caring for their family member with dementia in the month prior to institutionalisation. By contrast, home-care nurses provided 16 hours of care, and home help aides between one and two hours (Bergh et al., 2015). Caring for people with dementia is seen to be more difficult than for many people with physical disabilities. This can be due to a combination of factors including the more intensive supervision often needed by people with dementia, higher prevalence of depression among those with dementia, and difficulties with communication, including appreciation for the caregiver (Schulz and Sherwood, 2008). In addition, caregivers are often ill-prepared to respond to the progressive nature of the condition, and the growing number and increasing complexity of the needs of people with dementia. These challenges can further contribute to emotional strain and burn-out among caregivers.

Caregiver stress can impact the health outcomes of people with dementia

The physical and mental health impacts of caring for people with dementia are significant, and deserve attention and tailored interventions that can help to reduce the impact on the caregiver. But improving caregiver health is also important to the well-being of those they care for. Caregiver burden is an important determinant of early institutionalisation (D'Onofrio et al., 2014; Gallagher et al., 2011; Mittelman et al., 2006; Gaugler et al., 2009; Spillman and Long, 2009; Yaffe et al., 2002). Multiple studies suggest that higher caregiver stress increases the desire and likelihood to institutionalise care recipients with dementia. Beyond the broad category of "caregiver stress," financial difficulty, physical stress, social support, family cohesion and caregiver knowledge about dementia have been associated with higher desire and likelihood toward institutionalisation (Spitznagel et al., 2006; Spillman and Long, 2009). Caregiver burden and health have also been associated with worse health outcomes for their recipients of care. Caregivers of people with dementia with higher levels of burden, caring intensity, depression, and lower educational attainment have been found to report higher levels of behavioural and psychiatric symptoms of dementia (BPSD) among the people they care for (Sink et al., 2006). Higher caregiver burden has also been associated with a higher prevalence of falls among care recipients (Vaughon et al., 2018; Kuzuya et al., 2006). Researchers have suggested promoting interventions that reduce these and other sources of caregiver stress as a means of delaying institutionalisation and improving health outcomes among people with dementia.

3.4.2. OECD countries have developed a range of policies to improve caregiver well-being, but more needs to be done to increase the take-up and impact of these services

The political focus on improving caregiver outcomes has grown

With the impact of caring on both caregivers and recipients of care well established, countries have developed a range of interventions that aim to improve the quality of life for carers. In recent years, a number of countries have signalled their commitment to reducing the burden on caregivers through the development of national caregiver plans and strategies, including Australia, Ireland, and Norway. Many caregiver interventions, including these national plans and strategies, address caregivers broadly, rather than focusing specifically on those providing care for people with dementia. Virtually all countries with national dementia strategies and plans make explicit reference to improving conditions for informal carers, though the level of detail provided varies across countries. Austria's national dementia strategy, for example, identifies informal carers as an important target group of the strategy and calls for improved skill-building for informal carers. In Norway, the national dementia plan has integrated aspects of informal care policies outlined in the country's national care plan and focuses on improving support, respite and training for informal carers. Family carers are compensated by municipalities, who are responsible for long-term care (Colombo, F. et al., 2011). In England, the 2014 Care Act has enshrined new rights for informal carers, including a right to a needs assessment by the local authority, and the provision of subsequent support.

Countries have adopted a combination of dementia-specific and broad-based carer policies to improve caregiver outcomes. Broad caregiver policies including workplace legislation providing for (paid or unpaid) caregiver leave, flexible work arrangements, respite care, and government financial supports or carer subsidies. These policies do not need to be explicitly targeted to people living with dementia for them to make a substantial impact on the lives of those with dementia and their informal carers. Other interventions are much more targeted at people caring for family members or friends with dementia, including skill-building and training programmes and counselling and support groups.

Many countries have developed policies that protect working carers

The time invested in caring can be substantial, particularly when care recipients have dementia. For informal carers who are still working, the dual demands of formal employment and carer responsibilities are often at odds, and can put considerable strain on performing well in one or both. The population of informal carers who continue to work is substantial, with between 40 and 60% of informal carers in Australia participating in the labour force alongside caring (Bittman, Hill and Thomson, 2007). Even when informal carers remain employed, they earn less than non-carers with equivalent qualifications, suggesting that the flexibilities needed to provide care – particularly intensive care – may limit employment opportunities (Carmichael and Charles, 2003). As the intensity of caregiving increases, the proportion of informal carers employed in the formal labour market falls, an effect that is particularly pronounced for female carers (Bittman, Hill and Thomson, 2007, Carmichael and Charles, 2003). Many informal carers are family members – often spouses or children – of the people with dementia they care for, and may have previously contributed to the finances of the household. Providing informal care can displace at least some of the family's earnings and can lead to increased stress over finances, a major driver of caregiver stress (Spillman and Long, 2009). The rising role of women in the labour market and their growing contribution to household finances has further increased the opportunity cost of forgoing or reducing employment for informal care (Carmichael and Charles, 2003).

Policies that allow informal carers to take leave from their positions or adopt flexible work schedules can help them stay in the formal employment sector. Across the OECD, 27 countries have adopted policies that provide for leave to care for family members. In 19 of these countries, leave is paid for at least some of the time spent caring.

Table 3.3. Leave entitlements to care for sick or ill family members

Country	Leave for carers	Paid leave available
Australia	Yes	Yes
Austria	Yes	Yes
Belgium	Yes	Yes
Canada	Yes	Yes (for family members at risk of dying in next 26 weeks; for employees who have worked >=600 hours in past year))
Chile		
Czech Republic	Yes	Yes
Denmark		
Estonia	Yes	Yes
Finland	Yes	
France	Yes	Not remunerated by employer (except in certain cases with collective conventions)
Germany	Yes	Yes) (short-term carer grant available regardless of employer size)
Greece	Yes	
Hungary		
Iceland		
Ireland	Yes	Yes (for close family member, where employee has worked for >= 12 months)
Israel	Yes	Yes (for spouse or parent)
Italy	Yes	Yes
Japan	Yes	Yes
Korea	Yes	
Latvia		
Luxembourg		
Mexico		
Netherlands	Yes	Yes (though employers can refuse "on serious business grounds")
New Zealand	Yes	Yes (for employees who have worked for >='26' weeks)
Norway	Yes	
Poland	Yes	Yes
Portugal	Yes	
Slovak Republic	Yes	Yes
Slovenia	Yes	Yes (co-resident family members)
Spain	Yes	Yes (though employers can refuse on "serious business grounds")
Sweden	Yes	Yes
Switzerland	Yes	
Turkey		
United Kingdom	Yes	
United States	Yes	

Source: OECD Family Database 2016.

More than half of OECD countries (19 countries) offers leave entitlements for family carers that includes at least some period of paid leave. In most countries offering paid leave for informal carers, leave is paid for a limited duration, in most cases for less than two weeks, though unpaid leave is often much longer. Paid leave is also sometimes tied to the employee's sick leave allowance. Both Israel and New Zealand deduct the time spent caring for sick family members from the carer's own allotted sick leave. In the Netherlands and Spain, employers are allowed to refuse requests for care leave if there is a strong business cause for doing so. A number of countries have criteria based on employer size (Ontario Canada, the United States), or employment history (Canada, Ireland, New Zealand, the United States) that can exclude some carers from eligibility. Given the long duration of dementia, this short period of paid leave can be of limited help. Programmes that allow for more work flexibility, including reducing hours and teleworking, may be better suited in supporting carers of people with dementia over the longer-term. In the United Kingdom (England), for example, all employees – including carers – may request to have a flexible working arrangement after an initial 26 week qualifying period. In Germany, a family care leave scheme was recently introduced to support employees needing to support a relative requiring long-term care. Employees may take up to six months off of work full-time, or elect to work part-time for up to 24 hours. Three months of leave is provided when caring for relatives at the end of life. In addition to the leave provided, employees have the opportunity to access interest-free loans (conditional on employer size) to help support them while their income is reduced. Respite care is available in some countries, but is often limited by local capacity constraints.

In addition to policies developed to support the livelihoods and financial stability of caregivers and their families, interventions that support the caregiver's own personal well-being can improve the quality of life of both carers and the people they care for. Respite care, which is designed to offer caregivers a break from their regular caregiving duties, is regularly cited as an important component of support for caregivers. Some respite care services are designed to offer short-term, often regular breaks in care. These often included day care services delivered through municipalities and community organisations, or in-home care services. In addition to such day services, some countries offer caregivers the opportunity to take longer breaks in caring by offering temporary placements in residential care services, such as local nursing homes. Emergency respite care services, which offer caregivers respite services on short notice, are less regularly available, though a number of countries have recognised the need to develop these programmes further. As with policies supporting caregiver livelihoods, most respite care services are not offered specifically for caregivers of people living with dementia, but are available more broadly to people living in the community with an assessed level of need.

While many countries report to have overnight respite care services, its availability can vary greatly by municipality or local community. In some countries, including Norway, Denmark, Ireland and Sweden, respite care is determined based on need, and recommended or prescribed as part of the personalised care plan developed in concert with case managers. In Austria, respite care is available as part of social care supports for informal carers, and must be applied for. Because of the high cost of providing respite services, some countries have determined legal maximums for the number of days carers may receive overnight respite care services. In New Zealand, respite care is funded to a maximum of 28 days per year, while in Israel, no more than two weeks are reimbursed.

Few countries have made access to overnight respite care a right for informal carers, though Germany offers a legal entitlement to a minimum number of respite care and short-term care days per year. Families can be reimbursed for up to six weeks of respite and short-term care per year. To provide financial stability to families, cash allowances for caregivers continue to be paid (at 50%) even when carers are using respite or short-term care services.

Overnight respite care is commonly provided by offering temporary residence in local nursing homes or other long-term care institutions. Many municipalities have developed agreements with local nursing homes to use a designated number of beds for respite care, though the availability can vary substantially by community. Innovative respite care services that promote carer relaxation while also integrating activities for people with dementia have also been developed. In Austria, a holiday respite care programme for people with dementia and their families integrates external care for people with dementia and training for carers into a holiday for the family. Carers are able to enjoy a break from their caregiving duties in a holiday setting without being fully removed from the person they care for, allowing them to relax without as much worry about the conditions of the person they normally care for as had they left them in a residential care setting (WHO, 2012).

Day care services are available, though they are not always dementia-specific and uptake can be low

Many OECD countries have developed day services that are exclusively available for people living with dementia. While Alzheimer's Disease International has published a guide to developing community-based day care centres, most countries have not developed guidelines or other recommendations related to day care for people living with dementia. Dementia-specific day programmes are often run by nongovernmental organisations, notably national Alzheimer's Associations, though in some countries – including New Zealand and Sweden – dementia-specific programmes are offered through local government services and can require a formal diagnosis of dementia for attendance. Day care services and programmes can vary significantly between centres. In Israel, day centre services are offered by the Ministry of Welfare and multiple non-governmental agencies, including the Israel Alzheimer's Association. In Sweden, day care is the most common form of non-medical support for people with dementia and is integrated into the care pathway. Case managers recommend day care as part of their individualised care plan, and day centre facilities then report back to case managers about how these plans are being followed. Day care is similarly recommended by case managers or care co-ordinators in other countries, including Ireland and Norway.

In many countries, uptake of day care services is strong, with some countries reporting that available services are oversubscribed. A 2009 review of available day care services in Greece found that demand for day care far exceeded available supply, with only about 5 000 people attending day care centres and many more on waiting lists for admission. Even in countries where day services are available, they can be geographically concentrated, particularly around cities. In New Zealand, both dementia-specific day centres and general day care programmes are offered throughout the country, though important gaps in coverage persist in rural areas of the country.

Across the OECD, day care services are the most widely available form of respite care for people living with dementia and their carers. Day care services can offer clear benefits to the person living with dementia. They often provide an important source of social interaction and stimulating activities for people with dementia, who would otherwise spend the majority of their time at home. The role of day centres as a form of respite for carers may not be their primary purpose at all. In contrast, longer-term respite care services, in which people with dementia are temporarily placed in residential care, can be more directly linked to relieving the burden on caregivers, though they can also serve as a 'test' period to evaluate how someone will do in institutional care. In Chile, the role of community-based day care centres is an integral pillar of the country's national plan on dementia. Notably, it strongly emphasises the role of informal carers in community-based care, going so far as to require people with dementia to be partnered with a caregiver in order to access services. This is only the second plan in Chile – after services for childbirth – that requires the participation of more than the direct patient (Box 3.5).

In many communities, demand for day care services, particularly those tailored to people with dementia, is high. However, in others participation rates have been reported to be very low. This raises questions about why in some circumstances, available services are not being fully utilised. This is especially perplexing given that in assessments of carer needs, carers frequently cite the availability of respite care as one of the most desired support services (Leong et al., 2001, Neville et al., 2015). In Switzerland, for example, the supply of day centre places much exceeds current levels of demand. This raises questions over what barriers might be keeping informal carers from accessing available services. Barriers in information and awareness of available services, negative connotations about respite care, and concerns about poor quality compared to self-delivered care have been cited in literature on respite care as possible obstacles to increasing the use of available services (Neville et al., 2015, Ashworth and Baker, 2000). In addition, financial and physical access barriers should be considered when developing day care services. In some circumstances, short day schedules and a lack of transportation services may preclude working carers from using available day centres. In Lucerne, Switzerland, local day centres have developed a full service around day centre activities. Staff from the day centres comes to the home of participating persons, helping them to get ready for the day and driving them to and from the day care centre. These options can give informal carers more flexibility to send their family members to available care where their schedules might otherwise not have allowed. Providing transportation and other linking services may be particularly important in rural areas, where the distances to available services may be considerable. In a previous qualitative study from Scotland, transportation and the effort to get family members with dementia ready to leave the house were cited as major barriers to accessing available services (Innes et al., 2005). Given the range of respite care services and activities, the obstacles to greater uptake are likely highly context-specific. Where uptake of available day care and other community services is low, communities should evaluate the needs of informal carers in the area to better understand how such programmes could be better tailored to meet their needs.

People who care for friends or family members with dementia will nearly always need some form of training or skill-building support to help them prepare for their new role. In recent years, a strong body of evidence – including a number of randomised control trials – has emerged for the effectiveness of caregiver training and skill-building interventions on caregiver burden, stress levels, and quality of care delivered (Gitlin et al., 2015). Individual behaviour management therapy to help caregivers respond to behavioural problems has been found to help reduce depression among caregivers for a sustained period, while caregivers who had received training on coping strategies was also found to reduce psychological distress (Selwood et al., 2007). A wide range of pilot interventions to improve caregivers outcomes have been identified in recent literature, with at least seven meta-analyses and 17 systematic reviews conducted in recent years, with more than 200 caregiver interventions identified as effective (Gitlin et al., 2015). Indeed, a major gap identified by researchers appears to be the delay in translating established research findings into broader policy interventions that reach caregivers in need of support.

Box 3.5. Developing integrated community-based day care centres for people with dementia in Chile

The Kintun model of community-based dementia care offers an informative example of how multiple services can be effectively integrated to deliver care that promotes community participation for both people with dementia and their carers. Despite a relatively high income per capita, large health inequalities persist throughout Chile, and few services currently exist to support people with dementia and their family carers (Gajardo et al., 2017). Indirect costs for dementia care – largely attributable for informal care – have been estimated to comprise 75% of the total cost of dementia in Chile, with caregiver burden particularly high among people of lower socioeconomic status (Hojman et al., 2017). Social costs account for just 5% of costs (Hojman et al., 2017).

Starting in 2013, the National Service for the Elderly launched a pilot project in the municipality of Penalolen that aimed to improve the independence of community-dwelling people with dementia (Kardish, 2014). The programme was designed around the concept of day-care centres for the elderly, but offers services – through day care, case management, home visits, and training for carers – that are more highly specialised and targeted toward people living with dementia than general day services. Five major components define the programme, which is open to residents of the municipality who are over the age of 60, participate in the public healthcare system, have a carer over 18, and who have been diagnosed with mild to moderate dementia:

Comprehensive geriatric assessment: The initial geriatric assessment identifies unmet needs and individual care plans are developed together with the person with dementia's family.

Day care: Day care services are offered once to twice per week and are designed to offer respite for family caregivers while offering people with dementia social interaction and stimulation. Individual groups are limited to fewer than 17 participants, and activities are developed based on the abilities of the group and their personal backgrounds. In order to facilitate participation, the day care services include transportation to and from the care centre and daytime meals.

Home visits: People with dementia receive at least one home visit as part of the Kintun programme. The home visit provides information to families on the skills needed to care for people living with dementia in their own homes, including reducing risks.

Caregiver training: Participants in the Kintun programme who have dementia must participate with a family carer. Family carers must commit to a minimum of two training sessions, which address caregiver readiness and response to difficult situations and link caregivers to available resources and support services in the community.

Case management: Participants receive case management to help them through different components related to the programme. Broader case management, for help with health and social services beyond the Kintun programme, is not offered.

The day care programme offered through Kintun is tailored specifically toward people with dementia, and includes activities related to cognitive function and social and community interaction. Many of the chosen programme components connect in some way to culturally significant activities. Exercise and social interaction, including with the broader community through activities such as gardening and museum visits, are also valued. Initial evaluation results of the Kintun programme suggest that while there are no cognitive benefits, there were reductions in falls, improvements in the behavioural and psychological symptoms of dementia, and improvements in how carers perceived people with dementia living at home (Aravena et al., 2017a; Aravena et al., 2017b). Based on the success of the initial Kintun community centre, the Ministry of Health began supporting the programme in 2015, with plans to build another nine centres across Chile in the next two years.

Nearly all OECD countries interviewed for this analysis reported that caregiver training and support programmes are available following a dementia diagnosis. Frequently offered caregiver interventions include short-term community-based training programmes, online training support tools, and in-person community support groups for families and carers of people with dementia. In the majority of cases, these programmes are primarily delivered by the nongovernmental sector, with Alzheimer's Associations and other dementia organisations playing a substantial role in the organisation and delivery of post-diagnostic caregiver support. In New Zealand, for example, Alzheimer's New Zealand and Dementia New Zealand both provide support groups and basic training seminars, run largely on a voluntary basis, to provide information on behaviour management, recognising symptoms, and information about the life course of dementia.

Caregiver-directed training and counselling is less frequently offered through government services, though where such programmes have been initiated, evaluations on their impact and cost-effectiveness have sometimes been encouraging. In the United States, the Resources for Enhancing Alzheimer's Caregiving Health (REACH) intervention was implemented across the Department of Veterans Affairs following the positive impact demonstrated by the programme in a randomised controlled trial conducted by the National Institute on Ageing an National Institute of Nursing Research (Nichols et al., 2011; Nichols et al., 2017). In addition to the VA, REACH has been incorporated into the U.S. Indian Health Service (IHS) and many states' Alzheimer's and dementia plans.

3.4.3. Countries are beginning to recognise the importance of measuring outcomes for carers

Improving the effectiveness of policies that support carers of people with dementia relies on the effectiveness of existing policies being measurable. The BeACCoN Network in Canada recently undertook a project that aimed to understand what data on caregivers is measured in OECD countries. This work, which included a literature review and national policy interviews with seven OECD countries (Australia, Canada, Ireland, Spain, Sweden, the United Kingdom, the United States) on caregiver issues, suggests that while some countries have begun to develop caregiver outcome measures, data on carers is not well developed in OECD countries.

National-level data on carers has begun to be collected in some OECD countries, including Australia, Canada, the United Kingdom and the United States. These data are often collected by government statistical agencies, such as the Australian Bureau of Statistics or the Office of National Statistics in the United Kingdom, but may also collected by NGOs, such as the Change Foundation in Canada, Carers UK in the United Kingdom or the National Alliance for Caregiving in the United States.

Existing measures focus mostly on outcomes with fewer relating to experiences and costs

Health systems across OECD countries have increasingly adopted measurement frameworks that address multiple factors, including patient outcomes, experience, and costs. Results from a literature review and interviews conducted between the BeACCoN network and national policymakers indicate that the majority of current measurement is focused on outcomes, with fewer measures available for experiences and costs.

Table 3.4. Carer measurement tools

Domain	Measurement tool	Components measured
Outcomes		Stigma, physical and mental health, role, hours spent caregiving, burden, depression/anxiety
	Australian National Survey Tool Called ABC123	• Physical health • Hours spent caring • Caregiver burden
	Household, Income and Labour Dynamics in Australia (HILDA); the Families Caring for a Person with Disability Study (FCPDS); Australian Bureau of Statistics' (ABS) Survey of Disability, Ageing and Carers	• Emotional health • Socio-demographic characteristics • Amount of face-to-face social contact • Fall-back carer • Financial assistance • Respite care • Emotional support • Physical health • Need for more support
Experiences		Approaches to carer support, the rights of family carers, services and their co-ordination, patterns of formal service use with informal care, experiences of care transitions
	National Background Reports (NABAREs) – describes the current situation of family carers in 23 EU countries	• Approaches to carer support • The rights of family carers and their financial recognition • Services for family carers
Costs		Financial recognition of carers, cost of caregiving, income support, overall amount of money spent, amount reduced from paid work, type of out of pocket expenses
	Statistics Canada General Social Survey on Caregiving and Care Receiving	• Incurred caregiving expenses (not reimbursed) i.e. dwelling modifications, prescription and non-prescription drugs • Amount spent over the year (not reimbursed) • Total median amount spent • Finances over the past 12 months i.e. borrowed money, depleted savings, changed spending habits

Box 3.6. Measuring carer outcomes, experiences and costs: The case of Australia

The Australian Bureau of Statistics conducts a survey of ' Disability, Ageing and Carers' which collects data from people aged 60 and over, people with disabilities and their carers. This is a national survey that collects data on carer outcomes and experiences including demographics of carers, who carers provide care for, what their caregiving involves, what the impact of caring is, and patterns of formal service use with informal care.

The Australian Government Department of Families, Housing, Community Services and Indigenous Affairs use numerous surveys of young carers in Australia. These surveys include the Census of Population and Housing (2006), Survey of Disability, Ageing, and Carers (2003), and Household, Income and Labour Dynamics in Australia (HILDA) survey. These surveys cover carer outcomes, experiences, and costs. These include measuring hidden carers, duties of carers, income support, free time, emotional impact of caring, benefits of caring, post-school education, training and labour market participation.

The Mental Health Carers Report by the Mental Health Council of Australia conducts a survey of 50 questions specifically aimed towards carers of people with mental health issues. This survey covers carer's outcomes, experiences and costs including mental and physical health, perceived communication with clinicians, insufficient recovery-based care, and quality of staff.

A non-profit organisation, Carers Australia New South Wales (NSW), conducted a survey in 2016 which collected from carers information on **outcomes, experiences and costs** including health and well-being, employment, finances, service access, and unmet needs.

Four of fourteen countries reported measuring the costs of informal caregiving. One example of this is from an Australian study which included a quantitative analysis of existing national data sets to assess income support for carers, in addition to labour market participation (Commonwealth of Australia, 2009). As well, in Canada, a report by Statistics Canada reported on the financial and professional consequences of being a carer and out-of-pocket costs which included transportation, medication, rehabilitation, overall amount spent, amount reduced from paid work, and type of support (Turcotte, 2013).

Few countries reported that caregiver experience is regularly measured. In some cases, regional-level planning bodies incorporated caregiver experience into their measurement systems. In Ontario, Canada, for example, the Local Health Integration Networks (LHINs) collect information on caregiver experience related to home and community care services. This information is used to provide the home care sector with quantitative data that can be used to compare patient's experiences when they receive services and to help the home care sector determine where more work is needed (Health Quality Ontario, 2017). In Australia, the Survey of Disability, Ageing and Carers (SDAC) is a continuous survey which was conducted over various time periods from 1981-2009 and since 2009 has been conducted every three years. This survey collects information on carer experiences including what activities carers assisted with and the relationship between carer and care recipient. This information is used to measure prevalence of disability across the country and to provide demographic and socio-economic data on those with disabilities, older adults, and their carers. This data can then be compared to the general population and used to estimate the number of carers for those with disabilities and over the age of 65, while also gathering more in-depth information about these carers (Australian Bureau of Statistics, 2017).

One of the areas of measurement that is particularly lacking is the positive impact of caregiving. Through the environmental scan, only Australia measured the positive benefits of caregiving. One report from Australia specifically looked at the positive benefits of young carers including being proud, strengthening the bond with family members, and gaining caring skills (Commonwealth of Australia, 2009). Carers have cited that caregiving resulted in feeling companionship, fulfilment or reward, and enjoyment (Cohen et al., 2002). These carers who reported positive feelings were less likely to experience negative outcomes including depression, burden, or poor health (Cohen et al., 2002). Caregiver participants in a workshop held by the BeACCoN research network also emphasised that the positive aspects of caregiving should be considered in carer-reported measures.

Most measures for carers are self-reported and collected through surveys, but the timeliness of this data is not always sufficient for use in policy-making

Many of the outcomes that are important to carers, including their quality of life or mental health, are best measured by asking the carers themselves. Correspondingly, most of the data that has been collected on carers is self-reported through surveys. Surveys are often run nationally through statistics agencies and other governmental bodies, though regular surveys can also be run by NGOs. For example, Carers UK has developed a carer-specific survey that includes 70 questions asking about a range of factors, from the support that people receive to whether they are able to pay their utility bills.

In some countries (Australia, Canada, Finland, Ireland and the United Kingdom) surveys exist that target carers specifically. In Australia, for example the Australian Bureau of Statistics collects data on a range of variables including location, age, whether the carer is the primary caregiver, information on the care recipient's condition, housing, and other factors. They also collect information about care recipient needs, such as activities of daily living (ADLs). In England, the National Health Service (NHS) conducts a specific household survey that includes caregiver measures such as who they are caring for, services provided, and health impacts of unpaid care, while local authorities in England are also required to survey carer quality of life. In this survey, carers are asked about the care recipient: i.e. parents, children, etc. Other groups such as non-governmental organisations (NGOs) collect data and do comparisons by age and other population level variables. These groups collect data on variables such as life satisfaction, psychological distress, and employment. For example, the National Alliance for Caregiving in the United States conducted an Online Caregiving in the US survey and collected data on: Experience, Outcome, and Costs. This included prevalence of carers in the US, demographic characteristics, financial burden of carers, nature of carer activities, and carer stress, strain, and health.

While the information collected through national surveys can be comprehensive, the timeliness of the data means it cannot always be used to regularly inform policymaking. In Spain, for example, the National Institute of Statistics conducts a comprehensive survey called 'The Primary Caregivers Questionnaire'. This questionnaire obtains very detailed information on caregiving and allows for comparisons on gender and outcomes such as health status. It also looks at frequency, intensity and duration of care, types of tasks performed, and the relationship between carer and care recipient. It then also asks dichotomous questions about health status impact on professional or economic life leisure, social life family life, or personal care. Though comprehensive, the survey is conducted only every ten years. This makes it difficult to measure how policy changes may affect caregiver experience and outcomes.

A similar challenge can be seen where census data is used for caregiver measurement. The 2011 census in the United Kingdom asked the whole population whether and the intensity with which they provide unpaid support alongside questions about ethnicity, faith, employment, gender, and health status. However, the next census will not be conducted until March 2021, which limits the usefulness of this data in assessing caregiver policy.

Surveys that collect data on a representative subset of the population can be run more frequently. Surveys of ageing, such as the Survey of Health, Ageing and Retirement in Europe (SHARE), the English Longitudinal Study of Ageing (ELSA) and the Health and Retirement Study (HRS) in the United States ask questions about the provision and receipt of informal care. Data are collected roughly every two years for people aged over 50.

Box 3.7. Different measuring bodies looking at carer measures

Canada – Collects data nationally via Statistics Canada and the Health Council of Canada surveys, regionally such as through Local Health Integration Networks (LHINs) and by the health regulator, Health Quality Ontario in Ontario, and advocacy groups such as the Change Foundation

Australia – Collects data from the Australian Bureau of Statistics, the Australian Institute, and NGOs

United States – Collects data through The Office of the Assistant Secretary for Planning and Evaluation, US Department of Health and Human Services; the National Alliance for Caregiving; the AARP Public Policy Institute; and, the United Hospital Fund

United Kingdom – Collects data via the Office for National Statistics; NGOs such as CarersUK; AgeUK; Dementia UK; Independent Age; Carers Trust; by region such as the Powys Carer Service and, Children's Commissioner for Wales; ICHOM

The outcome measures used in research are not always reflected in systematic data collections

In addition to nationally-collected survey data used to assess carers, a variety of carer measurement tools have been developed that are used primarily in research contexts. In academic research, scales such as the Carer Quality of Life, Zarit Burden Index, Carer Strain Index, Subjective Burden Scale, and Burden Scale for Family Caregivers. are often applied. The Adult Carer Quality of Life Questionnaire helps researchers or practitioners who have contact with carers. It assesses the quality of life of unpaid carers and can be used once or as a pre and post if testing the effects of a support or intervention (Elwick et al., 2010). The Zarit Burden Index is a carer self-report measure addressing mostly the personal and role strain of the carer (American Psychological Association, 2017). The Caregiver Strain Index is used to look at the subjective perceptions of the caretaking relationships by caregivers and the emotional health of caregivers (Robinson 1983). The Burden Scale for

Family Caregivers is a tool used to assess subjective burden of carers in a very short time frame (Graessel et al., 2014).

While these research scales offer an important level of depth in evaluating carers, they are not systematically used by either government or non-governmental agencies outside of academia. This may be due to cost. For example, the Family Caregivers Support Agreement tool is used to assess support needs for carers providing care for relatives at home – however it must be purchased to be used (Evaloris). Also, the Zarit Burden Index must be purchased depending upon the type of study using it, for example non-funded academic users (i.e. individual medical practice) can use it for free, but funded academic research (i.e. projects being funded by industry, government, EU or charities) and commercial users (i.e. industry or for-profit) must pay to use the tool (MAPI Research Trust, 2017). Carer agencies and organisations have in some cases developed their own surveys and methods, which could imply a lack of appropriate tools for carer measurement. There is inconsistency of use in the different types of scales and it appears that many organisations are developing their own that are less academic and more able to measure what is actually important for carers. Future work should assess the usability and applicability of these tools to broader, non-academic contexts.

Box 3.8. Carer measurement in the United Kingdom and Australia

Australia – Many organisations in Australia are collecting data regarding carers including Australian Institute of Health and Welfare and the Australian Government Department of Health and Ageing; Australian Government Department of Families, Housing, Community Services, and Indigenous Affairs; Australian Institute of Family Studies and Australian Government Department of Families, Community Services and Indigenous Affairs, and Carers Australia NSW. Between this multitude of organisations, all aspects of the Triple Aim (outcomes, experiences and costs) are being measured.

United Kingdom – Many agencies are collecting information specific to different groups of carers (i.e. people aged 65 and over, carers and care recipients, and young carers). These agencies include CarersUK, AgeUK, DementiaUK, Office for National Statistics, Independent Age, Powys Carers Service, Children's Commissioner for Wales, and Carers Trust. Although mainly outcome and experiences data are collected – cost is also measured by some organisations.

From the promising examples in the Australia, the United Kingdom and other countries, comprehensive measurement of carer outcomes, experiences and costs is not out of reach and OECD countries would do well to look to member countries' experiences to consolidate and build upon.

Varying definitions of carers make cross-country comparisons difficult

The lack of a common definition for an informal carer across OECD countries can challenge international comparisons of caregiver well-being (Colombo, F. et al., 2011). Some countries limited the definition to include only those who provided assistance with a care recipient's basic activities of daily living (ADLs), for example, while other countries expanded the definition to include those who also provide assistance with a care recipient's instrumental activities of daily living (IADLs) (Colombo, F. et al., 2011). Moreover, some people may not consider themselves to be carers, even where they provide caregiving services (Colombo, F. et al., 2011). Standardising the concept of informal caring to the greatest extent possible could better enable comparisons across countries.

Box 3.9. Defining carers

How carers are defined varies widely across countries. In New Zealand, for example, informal carers are restricted to people who care for children and young persons (aged 25 and under). Other countries, including Ireland, the United Kingdom, and Spain use a much broader definition for informal carers, and consider both family members and friends to be caregivers so long as they provide help with care and are not paid to do so.

Who is considered a carer can even differ within one country depending on the context. For example, there may be an interest in a more inclusive definition to determine who would qualify for services such as training or education, whilst a more stringent definition may be called for when determining whether carers are eligible for tax credits. Examples of this variance were found in our interviews with stakeholders in the United Kingdom and Spain who reported there not being a single definition for carers and that it differed depending on the context. In Spain, some researchers address the issue of caring from a broader perspective, which considers the care provided to be life sustaining and means that almost all people must receive care throughout their lives at some point. Whereas, a more restrictive definition exists under the Spanish Dependency Act and the degree of dependency is decided upon by each region (or Autonomous Communities), which means that resources are allocated based on these different definitions of level of dependency of the care recipient. In the UK, they note that there are many differing definitions between community care, social care, the NHS, etc. Carers in the United Kingdom are also officially mentioned in pension legislation. In Canada, three federally-legislated tax credits are available for carers, each of which has different eligibility criteria. As of the 2017 tax season, the three credits will be streamlined into one 'Canada Caregiver Credit' to improve access to financial support for carers (Government of Canada, 2017).

In some cases, carer measurement tools have been developed that focus on only specific groups of carers. In the United Kingdom (Dementia UK), Australia (Dementia Centre for Research Collaboration), and Ireland (Care Alliance Ireland), for example, measurement tools were developed for carers of people with dementia. Dementia UK surveyed carers who had received services by the Admiral Nurses' who provide support to families living with dementia, they use these findings to guide the professional development of the Admiral Nurses by targeting those areas where carers did not feel as well supported (Maio, Botsford & Iliffe, 2016). Care Alliance Ireland along with the Alzheimer Society of Ireland pushed to have a National Dementia Strategy published in 2014, which they want to be used to improve supports for those living with dementia and their families (Care Alliance Ireland, 2015). Tools for carers of people with HIV and mental health issues were developed in Canada and Australia, respectively.

Linking data on carers to care recipients could lead to richer indicators

As measuring caregiver outcomes, experience, and costs become more common, countries should consider how caregiver measures can be best linked to data on their recipients of care. There may be privacy or confidentiality issues that must be addressed for the carer and care recipient's data to be linked. In addition, logistical or administrative issues can challenge linking two different individuals within a survey or a census.

Better linking data between the carer and care recipient could help improve how the caregiving relationship is understood. Until now, patients have largely been organised based on condition, under the assumption that their disease is the unifying factor for providing services or support. However, there is a growing understanding, that segmentation based on condition is not sufficient to design or tailor care (Hostetter & Klein, 2015). Different health systems have begun to develop new ways to segment patients (Hostetter & Klein, 2015). Some health care systems are using segmentation to look for missing patients who do not seek care, while others are segmenting based on the values of patients or based on geography (Hostetter & Klein, 2015). Moreover, cultural or societal factors that differ between countries and within communities can influence how people seek and receive care. Carer's needs may sometimes be linked by the condition of the person they care for. But at other times, other factors – such as the carer's age, where they live, or their relationship to the person they care for – will play a larger role in their caregiving experience. Linking patients and their carers will facilitate a better understanding of how both carers and their recipients of care interact with and experience health and care services.

References

Aguirre, E. et al. (2013), "Cognitive stimulation therapy (CST) for people with dementia-who benefits most?", *International Journal of Geriatric Psychiatry*, Vol. 28, No. 3, pp. 284–290. https://doi.org/10.1002/gps.3823

Aihara, Y. et al. (2016), "Public attitudes towards people living with dementia: A cross-sectional study in urban Japan (innovative practice)", *Dementia*, Vol. 0, No. 0, pp. 1–9. https://doi.org/10.1177/1471301216682118.

Algar, K., Woods, R. T. and G. Windle (2016), "Measuring the quality of life and well-being of people with dementia: A review of observational measures", *Dementia*, Vol. 15, No. 4, pp. 832–857. https://doi.org/10.1177/1471301214540163-

Alzheimer's Australia (2014), *Dementia Care in the acute hospital setting: issues and strategies* [report], Alzheimer's Australia, Canberra.

Alzheimer's Disease International (2015), "Dementia Friendly Communities (DFCs)", Alzheimer's Disease International, London.

Alzheimer Europe (2017), *European Dementia Monitor 2017: Comparing and benchmarking national dementia policies and strategies*, Alzheimer Europe Report.

Alzheimer's Scotland (2017), *Alzheimer's Scotland Post – Diagnostic Support Campaign*, https://www.alzscot.org/news_and_community/news/4002_alzheimer_scotland_post-diagnostic_support_campaign.

Alzheimer's Disease International (2017), *Dementia Friends*, [website]. https://www.alz.co.uk/dementia-friendly-communities/dementia-friends

American Psychological Association (2017), "Zarit Burden Interview – Construct: Caregiver Burden", http://www.apa.org/pi/about/publications/caregivers/practice-settings/assessment/tools/zarit.aspx.

Andel, R. et al. (2008), "Physical exercise at midlife and risk of dementia three decades later: a population-based study of Swedish twins", *The Journals of Gerontology*, Series A, Biological Sciences and Medical Sciences. Vol. 63, No. 1, pp. 62-66.

Aravena, J. M. and J. Gajardo (2017), "The Kintun Program: Lessons for the Design of Activities for Persons with Dementia in Chile", *Innovation in Aging*, Vol. 1, No. S1, pp. 980–980. https://doi.org/10.1093/geroni/igx004.3539.

Aravena, J. M., Gajardo, J. and M. Budinich (2017), "The Kintun Program in Chile: Effects in Older Persons with Mild to Moderate Dementia", *Innovation in Aging*, Vol. 1, No. S1, pp. 162–163.

Ashworth, M. and A.H. Baker (2000), "'Time and space": carers" views about respite care", *Health & Social Care in the Community*, Vol. 8, No. 1, pp. 50–56.

Beerens, H.C. et al. (2014), "Quality of life and quality of care for people with dementia receiving long term institutional care or professional home care: The European RightTimePlaceCare Study", *The Journal of Post-Acute and Long-Term Care Medicine*, Vol. 15, No. 1, pp. 54-61.

Bergh, S. et al. (2015), "Resource use and disease course in dementia (short version)", Ressursbruk og sykdomsforløp ved demens (REDIC).

Bittman, M., Hill, T. and C. Thomson (2007), "The Impact of Caring on Informal Carers' Employment, Income and Earnings: a Longitudinal Approach", *Australian Journal of Social Issues*, Vol. 42, No. 2, pp. 255–272.

Bundesamtes für Gesundheit (Switzerland) (2017), "Nationale Demenzstrateegie: Teilprojekt 3.2 «Förderung der Koordination von Leistungen zur Deckung des individuellen Versorgungsbedarfs» 2014–2017", Bern.

Burton, L. C. et al. (2003), "Transitions in Spousal Caregiving," *The Gerontologist*, Vol. 43, No. 2, pp. 230–241.

Cannuscio, C. C. et al. (2002), "Reverberations of Family Illness: A Longitudinal Assessment of Informal Caregiving and Mental Health Status in the Nurses' Health Study", *American Journal of Public Health*, Vol. 92, No. 8, pp. 1305–1311. https://doi.org/10.2105/AJPH.92.8.1305.

Care Alliance Ireland (2015), "Family Caring in Ireland: Guiding support for family carers", http://www.carealliance.ie/userfiles/file/Family%20Caring%20in%20Ireland%20Pdf.pdf.

Carmichael, F. and S. Charles (2003), "The opportunity costs of informal care: does gender matter?", *Journal of Health Economics*, Vol. 22, No. 5, pp. 781–803. https://doi.org/10.1016/S0167-6296(03)00044-4

Chiu, H. F. K. et al. (2014), "Renaming dementia – an East Asian perspective", *International Psychogeriatrics*, Vol. 26, No. 6, pp. 885–887. https://doi.org/10.1017/S1041610214000453

Cohen, C.A., Colantonio, A. and L. Vernich (2002), "Positive aspects of caregiving: rounding out the caregiver experience", *International Journal of Geriatric Psychiatry*, Vol. 17, 184-188. https://doi.org/110.1002/gps.561.

Colombo, F. et al. (2011), *Help Wanted?: Providing and Paying for Long-Term Care*, OECD Health Policy Studies, OECD Publishing, Paris, http://dx.doi.org/10.1787/9789264097759-en.

Commonwealth of Australia (2009), "Young carers in Australia: understanding the advantages and disadvantages of their care giving", Social policy research paper No.38. https://www.dss.gov.au/sites/default/files/documents/05_2012/sprp_38.pdf.

D'Amico, F. et al. (2015), "Maintenance Cognitive Stimulation Therapy: An Economic Evaluation Within a Randomized Controlled Trial", *Journal of the American Medical Directors Association*, Vol. 16, No. 1, pp. 63–70. https://doi.org/10.1016/j.jamda.2014.10.020.

D'Onofrio, G. et al. (2014), "Caregiver burden characterization in patients with Alzheimer's disease or vascular dementia", *International Journal of Geriatric Psychiatry*, Vol. 30, pp. 891-899. https://doi.org/10.1002/gps.4232.

Department of Health. (2016). Prime Minister's Challenge on Dementia 2020: Implementation Plan.

Donnelly, L. (2014), "Businesses sign up 400,000 dementia friends", The Telegraph, 30 March 2014.

Douglas, A., Letts, L. and J. Richardson (2011), "A systematic review of accidental injury from fire, wandering and medication self-administration errors for older adults with and without dementia", *Archives of Gerontology and Geriatrics*, Vol. 52, No. 1, pp. e1–e10. https://doi.org/10.1016/j.archger.2010.02.014.

Elwick, H. et al. (2010), Manual for the Adult Carer Quality of Life Questionnaire (AC-QoL)", London: The Princess Royal Trust for Carers. Retrieved from: http://static.carers.org/files/adult-carer-qol-published-version-5571.pdf.

Etters, L., Goodall, D. and B. Harrison (2008), "Caregiver burden among dementia patient caregivers: A systematic review", *Journal of the American Association of Nurse Practitioners*, Vol. 20, No. 8. https://doi.org/10.1111/j.1745-7599.2008.00342.x.

Evaloris (n.d.). "Family Caregivers Support Agreement (FCSA) training kit", Retrieved from: https://evalorix.com/boutique/innovations-en-sante/family-caregivers-support-agreement-fcsa-kit/.

Fereshtehnejad, S.-M. et al. (2014), "Dementia diagnosis, treatment and care in specialist clinics in two scandinavian countries: a data comparison between the swedish dementia registry (svedem) and the danish dementia registry", *Alzheimer's & Dementia*, Vol. 10,, pp. P223–P224. https://doi.org/10.1016/j.jalz.2014.04.312.

Forbes, D. et al. (2015), "Exercise programs for people with dementia", *The Cochrane Database of Systematic Reviews*, Vol. 15, No. 4, https://doi.org/110.1002/14651858.CD006489.pub4.

Gajardo, J. et al. (2017), "The Kintun program for families with dementia: From novel experiment to national policy (innovative practice)", *Dementia*, Vol. 0, No. 0, pp. 1–8. https://doi.org/10.1177/1471301217721863.

Gallagher, D. et al. (2011), "Determinants of the desire to institutionalize in Alzheimer's caregivers", *American Journal of Alzheimer's Disease & Other Dementias*, Vol. 26, No. 3, pp. 205-211.

Gaugler, J. E. et al. (2009), "Predictors of Nursing Home Admission for Persons with Dementia", *Medical Care*, Vol. 47, No. 2, pp. 191–198.

Gitlin, L. N. et al. (2015), "Translating Evidence-Based Dementia Caregiving Interventions into Practice: State-of-the-Science and Next Steps", *The Gerontologist*, Vol. 55, No. 2, pp. 210–226. https://doi.org/10.1093/geront/gnu123.

Government of Canada. (2017), "Budget 2017: Chapter 4 – Tax fairness for the middle class", Retrieved from: http://www.budget.gc.ca/2017/docs/plan/chap-04-en.html.

Graessel, E. et al. (2014), "Subjective caregiver burden: validity of the 10-item short version of the Burden Scale for Family Caregivers BSFC-s", *BMC Geriatrics*, Vol. 14, No. 23. https://doi.org/10.1186/1471-2318-14-23.

Hostetter, M. and S. Klein (June 2015), "In Focus: Segmenting populations to tailor services, improve care", *Quality Matters Archive*. Retrieved from: http://www.commonwealthfund.org/publications/newsletters/quality-matters/2015/june/in-focus.

Maio, L., Botsford, J. and S. Iliffe (2016), "Family carers' experiences of the Admiral Nursing Service: a quantitative analysis of carer feedback", *Aging & Mental Health*, Vol. 20, No. 7, pp. 669-675. http://dx.doi.org/10.1080/13607863.2015.1052776 .

MAPI Research Trust (2017), "Zarit Burden Interview (ZBI)", Retrieved from: https://eprovide.mapi-trust.org/instruments/zarit-burden-interview#contact_and_conditions_of_use.

NHS National Services Scotland (2017), "Local Delivery Plan 2017/18 – 2021/22", Government of Scotland.

Hayashi, M. (2015), "Dementia: Japan's experience" (pp. 1–21). Presented at the Dementia Awareness Week Conference.

Hayashi, M. (2016), "Japan's journey towards age-friendly and dementia-friendly communities" (pp. 1–18). Presented at the Better Ageing in Japan and UK City Regions, Church House, Westminster.

Health Quality Ontario (2017), "Measuring Up 2017 – Technical Appendix", Retrieved from: http://www.hqontario.ca/Portals/0/documents/pr/measuring-up-technical-appendix-2017-en.pdf.

Heitmueller, A. and K. Inglis (2007), "The earnings of informal carers: wage differentials and opportunity costs", *Journal of Health Economics*, Vol. 26, No. 4, pp. 821-841.

Heward, M. et al. (2017), "Dementia-friendly communities: challenges and strategies for achieving stakeholder involvement", *Health & Social Care in the Community*, Vol. 25, No. 3, pp. 858–867. https://doi.org/10.1111/hsc.12371

Hirst, M. (2005), “Carer distress: A prospective, population-based study”, *Social Science & Medicine*, Vol. 61, No. 3, pp. 697–708. https://doi.org/10.1016/j.socscimed.2005.01.001.

Hoffmann, K. et al. (2016), “Moderate-to-High Intensity Physical Exercise in Patients with Alzheimer’s Disease: A Randomized Controlled Trial”, *Journal of Alzheimer's Disease*, Vol. 50, No. 2, pp. 443–453. https://doi.org/10.3233/JAD-150817

Hojman, D. A. et al. (2017), “The cost of dementia in an unequal country: The case of Chile”, *PLoS ONE*, Vol. 12, No. 3, pp. e0172204–17. https://doi.org/10.1371/journal.pone.0172204.

Hope, T. et al. (1994), “The Structure of Wandering in Dementia”, *International Journal of Geriatric Psychiatry*, Vol. 9, No. 2, pp. 149–155.

Hope T. et al. (2001), “Wandering in Dementia: A Longitudinal Study”, *International Psychogeriatrics*, Vol. 13, No. 2, pp. 137-147. https://doi.org/10.1017/S1041610201007542

Innes, A. et al. (2005), “Dementia care provision in rural Scotland: service users’ and carers’ experiences”, *Health & Social Care in the Community*, Vol. 13, No. 4, pp. 354–365.

International Cognitive Stimulation Therapy Centre (2017), “CST by country”, [website], International Cognitive Stimulation Therapy Centre, University College London, London. https://www.ucl.ac.uk/international-cognitive-stimulation-therapy/countries.

Jansen, A. P. D. et al. (2011), “Effectiveness of case management among older adults with early symptoms of dementia and their primary informal caregivers: A randomized clinical trial”, *International Journal of Nursing Studies*, Vol. 48, No. 8, pp. 933–943. https://doi.org/10.1016/j.ijnurstu.2011.02.004

Kardish, C. (2014), “Chile’s Deceptively Simple Dementia Care Model: Treat Patients Like Adults.” Retrieved August 28, 2017, from http://www.governing.com/topics/health-human-services/gov-chile-dementi-care-model.html.

Klein, D. A. et al. (1999), “Wandering behaviour in community-residing persons with dementia”, *International Journal of Geriatric Psychiatry*, Vol. 14, No. 4, pp. 272–279. https://doi.org/10.1002/(SICI)1099-1166(199904)14:4<272::AID-GPS896>3.0.CO;2-P

Koch, T. et al. (2012), “The potential of case management for people with dementia: a commentary”, *International Journal of Geriatric Psychiatry*, Vol. 27, No. 12, pp. 1305–1314. https://doi.org/10.1002/(ISSN)1099-1166.

Koike, S. et al. (2015), “Long-term effect of a name change for schizophrenia on reducing stigma”, *Social Psychiatry and Psychiatric Epidemiology*, Vol. 50, No. 10, pp. 1519–1526. https://doi.org/10.1007/s00127-015-1064-8.

Kuzuya, M. et al. (2006), “Falls of the elderly are associated with burden of caregivers in the community”, *International Journal of Geriatric Psychiatry*, Vol. 21, No. 8, pp. 740–745. https://doi.org/10.1002/gps.1554.

Larson, E. B. et al. (2006), “Exercise Is Associated with Reduced Risk for Incident Dementia among Persons 65 Years of Age and Older”, *Annals of Internal Medicine*, Vol. 144,, pp. 73–81.

Lautenschlager, N.T. et al. (2008), “Effect of physical activity on cognitive function in older adults at risk for Alzheimer disease: a randomized trial”, *Journal of the American Medical Association*, Vol. 300, No. 9, pp. 1027-1037. https://doi.org/10.1001/jama.300.9.1027.

Leong, J., Madjar, I., and B. Fiveash (2001), “Needs of Family Carers of Elderly People with Dementia Living in the Community”, *Australasian Journal on Ageing*, Vol. 20, No. 3, pp. 133–138.

Livingston, G. et al. (2017), "Dementia prevention, intervention, and care", *The Lancet*, Vol. 390, No. 10113, pp. 1–62. https://doi.org/10.1016/S0140-6736(17)31363-6.

Logsdon, R. G. et al. (1998), "Wandering: A Significant Problem Among Community Residing Individuals With Alzheimer's Disease", *Journal of Gerontology*, Vol. 53B, No. 5, pp. 294–299.

McShane, R., Areosa Sastre, A. and N. Minakaran (2006), "Memantine for dementia", *The Cochrane Database of Systematic Reviews*, Vol. 19, No. 2.

Ministry of Health (2013). *New Zealand Framework for Dementia Care*. Wellington: Ministry of Health.

Ministry of Health, Labour and Welfare (2017), "Establishing 'the Community-based Integrated Care System'", Ministry of Health, Labour and Welfare, Tokyo, Japan.

Mittelman, M. S. et al. (2006), "Improving caregiver well-being delays nursing home placement of patients with Alzheimer disease", *Neurology*, Vol. 67, No. 9, pp. 1592–1599. https://doi.org/10.1212/01.wnl.0000242727.81172.91.

Miyamoto, M., George, D. R. and P.J. Whitehouse (2011), "Government, professional and public efforts in Japan to change the designation of dementia (chiho)", *Dementia*, Vol. 10, No. 4, pp. 475–486. https://doi.org/10.1177/1471301211416616.

National Collaborating Centre for Mental Health, (2016). *A NICE-SCIE Guideline on supporting people with dementia and their carers in health and social care: National Clinical Practice Guideline Number 42*, The British Psychological Society & The Royal College of Psychiatrists, London.

Neville, C. et al. (2015), "Literature review: use of respite by carers of people with dementia", *Health & Social Care in the Community*, Vol. 23, No. 1, pp. 51–63. https://doi.org/10.1111/hsc.12095.

Nichols, L.O. et al. (2011), "Translation of a Dementia Caregiver Support Program in a Health Care System—REACH VA", *Archives of Internal Medicine*, Vol. 171, No. 4, pp. 353–359.

Nichols, L.O. et al. (2017), "Impact of the REACH II and REACH VA Dementia Caregiver Interventions on Healthcare Costs", *Journal of the American Geriatric Society*, Vol. 65, No. 5, pp. 931-936.

OECD (2016), *PF2.3: Additional leave entitlements for working parents*, OECD Family Database. http://www.oecd.org/els/family/database.htm.

OECD (2017), *Health at a Glance 2017: OECD Indicators*, OECD Publishing, Paris, http://dx.doi.org/10.1787/health_glance-2017-en.

Öhman, H. et al. (2016), "Effects of exercise on cognition: The Finnish Alzheimer Disease Exercise Trial: A Randomized, Controlled Trial", *Journal of the American Geriatrics Society*, Vol. 64, No. 4, pp. 731-738.

Orrell, M. et al. (2005), "A pilot study examining the effectiveness of maintenance Cognitive Stimulation Therapy (MCST) for people with dementia", *International Journal of Geriatric Psychiatry*, Vol. 20, No. 5, pp. 446–451. https://doi.org/10.1002/gps.1304.

Ory, M. G. et al. (1999), "Prevalence and Impact of Caregiving: A Detailed Comparison Between Dementia and Nondementia Caregivers", *The Gerontologist*, Vol. 39, No. 2, pp. 177–185.

Parker, D., Mills, S. and J. Abbey (2008), "Effectiveness of interventions that assist caregivers to support people with dementia living in the community: a systematic review", *International Journal of Evidence-Based Healthcare*, Vol. 6, pp. 137–172. https://doi.org/10.1111/j.1479-6988.2008.00090.x.

Peeters, J.M. et al. (2016), "Does the organisational model of dementia case management make a difference in satisfaction with case management and caregiver burden? An evaluation study", *BMC Geriatrics*, Vol. 16, No. 65. https://doi.org/10.1186/s12877-016-0237-y.

Perales, J. et al. (2013), "Health-related quality-of-life instruments for Alzheimer's disease and mixed dementia", *International Psychogeriatrics*, Vol. 25, No. 5, pp. 691-706, https://doi.org/10.1017/S1041610212002293.

Pharmaceutical Society of Australia. (2014), "Dementia", inPHARMation, Vol. 15, No. 6.

Pimouguet, C. et al. (2013), "The 2008-2012 French Alzheimer Plan: A Unique Opportunity for Improving Integrated Care for Dementia", *Journal of Alzheimer's Disease*, Vol. 34,, pp. 307–314. https://doi.org/10.3233/JAD-121648.

Pinquart, M. and S. Sörensen (2003), "Differences between caregivers and noncaregivers in psychological health and physical health: A meta-analysis.", *Psychology and Aging*, Vol. 18, No. 2, pp. 250–267. https://doi.org/10.1037/0882-7974.18.2.250.

Reuben, D. B. et al. (2013), "The University of California at Los Angeles Alzheimer's and Dementia Care Program for Comprehensive, Coordinated, Patient-Centered Care: Preliminary Data", *Journal of the American Geriatrics Society*, Vol. 61, No. 12, pp. 2214–2218. https://doi.org/10.1111/jgs.12562.

Robinson, B.C. (1983), "Validation of a Caregiver Strain Index", *Journal of Gerontology*, Vol. 38, No. 3, pp. 344-8. https://www.ncbi.nlm.nih.gov/pubmed/6841931.

Rolinski, M. et al. (2012), "Cholinesterase inhibitors for dementia with Lewy bodies, Parkinson's disease dementia and cognitive impairment in Parkinson's disease", *The Cochrane Database of Systematic Reviews*, Vol. 14, No. 3, https://doi.org/10.1002/14651858.CD006504.pub2.

Schulz, R. and P.R. Sherwood (2008), "Physical and Mental Health Effects of Family Caregiving", *American Journal of Nursing*, Vol. 108, No. 9 Supplement, pp. 23–27. https://doi.org/10.1097/01.NAJ.0000336406.45248.4c.

Selwood, A. et al. (2007), "Systematic review of the effect of psychological interventions on family caregivers of people with dementia", *Journal of Affective Disorders*, Vol. 101, No. 1-3, pp. 75–89. https://doi.org/10.1016/j.jad.2006.10.025.

Sink, K.M. et al. (2006), "Caregiver characteristics are associated with neuropsychiatric symptoms of dementia", *Journal of the American Geriatrics Society*, Vol. 45, No. 5, pp. 796-803.

Spillman, B.C. and S.K. Long (2009), "Does High Caregiver Stress Predict Nursing Home Entry?", *Inquiry*, Vol. 46, pp. 140–161.

Spitznagel, M. B. et al. (2006), "Psychosocial Predictors of Dementia Caregiver Desire to Institutionalize: Caregiver, Care Recipient, and Family Relationship Factors", *Journal of Geriatric Psychiatry and Neurology*, Vol. 19, No. 1, pp. 16–20. https://doi.org/10.1177/0891988705284713.

Stansfeld, S. et al. (2014), "Stressors and common mental disorder in informal carers – An analysis of the English Adult Psychiatric Morbidity Survey 2007", *Social Science & Medicine*, Vol. 120, pp. 190-198.

Suzuki, M. et al. (2004), "Behavioral and endocrinological evaluation of music therapy for elderly patients with dementia", *Nursing and Health Sciences*, Vol. 6, pp. 11–18.

Tan, Z. S., Jennings, L. and D. Reuben (2014), "Coordinated Care Management For Dementia In A Large Academic Health System", *Health Affairs*, Vol. 33, No. 4, pp. 619–625. https://doi.org/10.1377/hlthaff.2013.1294.

Thomas, G.P.A. et al. (2015), "Informal carers' health-related quality of life and patient experience in primary care: evidence from 195,364 carers in England responding to a national survey", *BMC Family Practice*, Vol. 16, No. 62. https://doi.org/10.1186/s12875-015-0277-y.

Turcotte, M. (2013), "Family caregiving: What are the consequences", retrieved from: http://www.statcan.gc.ca/pub/75-006-x/2013001/article/11858-eng.pdf.

Vaingankar, J.A. et al. (2016), "Care participation and burden among informal caregivers of older adults with care needs and associations with dementia", *International Psychogeriatrics*, Vol. 28, No. 2, pp. 221-231.

Van Mierlo, L. D. et al. (2014), "Towards personalized integrated dementia care: a qualitative study into the implementation of different models of case management", *BMC Geriatrics*, Vol. 14, No. 84, pp. 1–14. https://doi.org/10.1186/1471-2318-14-84.

Vaughon, W. et al. (2018), "Association between falls and caregiving tasks among informal caregivers: Canadian Community Health Survey Data", *Canadian Journal on Aging*, Vol. 37, No. 1, pp. 70-75, https://doi.org/10.1017/S0714980817000496.

Vickrey, B. G. et al. (2006), "The Effect of a Disease Management Intervention on Quality and Outcomes of Dementia Care", *Annals of Internal Medicine*, Vol. 145, No. 10, pp. 713–726.

Viitanen, T.K. (2005), "Informal elderly care and women's labour force participation across Europe", *ENEPRI Research Reports*, No. 13. https://doi.org/10.2139/ssrn.2012280.

Vroomen, J. et al. (2012), "Comparing Dutch Case management care models for people with dementia and their caregivers: The design of the COMPAS study", *BMC Health Services Research*, Vol. 12, No. 132, pp. 1–10. https://doi.org/10.1186/1472-6963-12-132.

Wimo, A. et al. (2011), "The economic impact of dementia in Europe in 2008-cost estimates from the Eurocode project", *International Journal of Geriatric Psychiatry*, Vol. 26, No. 8, pp. 825–832. https://doi.org/10.1002/gps.2610.

Woods, B. et al. (2012), "Cognitive stimulation to improve cognitive functioning in people with dementia", *The Cochrane Database of Systematic Reviews*, Vol. 15, No. 2. https://doi.org/10.1002/14651858.CD005562.pub2.

World Health Organization. (2012), "Dementia: a public health priority", WHO Press, World Health Organization, Geneva.

Yaffe, K. et al. (2002), "Patient and Caregiver Characteristics and Nursing Home Placement in Patients With Dementia", *The Journal of the American Medical Association*, Vol. 287, No. 16, pp. 2090–2098. https://doi.org/10.1001/jama.287.16.2090.

Chapter 4. Health and long-term care services for advanced dementia are poor

This chapter examines what countries are doing to provide better care for people with advanced forms of dementia, including in care facilities, hospitals, and at the end of life. It finds that the quality of care for people with advanced dementia is in many cases poor. Better measurement, including strengthened hospital coding and more regular monitoring of quality of care measures, is important to ensure that best practice policies are more routinely implemented, particularly in formal care settings.

The statistical data for Israel are supplied by and under the responsibility of the relevant Israeli authorities. The use of such data by the OECD is without prejudice to the status of the Golan Heights, East Jerusalem and Israeli settlements in the West Bank under the terms of international law.

Though many countries have increasingly focused on community-based care and ageing in place, people with dementia nevertheless require significant professional support. People living at home with moderate dementia may need at least occasional help with basic activities of daily living, such as washing, dressing, and preparing meals, while many with more advanced forms of the disease will also require more intensive care support, including full-time home health aides or nursing staff. Those living in nursing homes or other long-term facilities will rely even more intensively on professional care support. People with dementia, and particularly advanced dementia, often exhibit psychological and behavioural symptoms from the disease and may become agitated or otherwise difficult to manage, particularly when confronted with new situations or people. Caring for people with dementia, who in addition to behavioural challenges may be unable to communicate their desires or needs, can be particularly difficult. Basic training programmes for professional health and social care staff may not adequately prepare professional carers for the challenges of caring well for someone with dementia. Dementia-specific approaches that take a person-centred approach to caring are critical for ensuring people with dementia require high-quality care from professional care workers and in long-term care institutions.

4.1. Ensuring better facility-based care for people with dementia

Traditional long-term care settings are often ill-suited to caring for the needs of people with dementia, and countries should consider how existing facilities can be adapted and new facilities can be developed to better meet the needs of people living with dementia. People living with dementia often have unique care needs that can be ill-suited to the traditional model of institutional care. In recent years, a better understanding of their needs has led to a re-evaluation of traditional models of long-term institutional care. Emerging models, including small-scale living communities and 'dementia villages' provide a more community-based model of support, even within institutional care settings.

However, driving further improvements in the quality of care offered in long-term care facilities is hampered by persisting data constraints. Dementia remains grossly underdiagnosed among people living in care facilities, and almost no countries have good data on the prevalence of dementia in care facilities. Nevertheless, estimates suggest that a majority of nursing home residents have cognitive impairment and dementia. Studies in Europe (Sweden, Czech Republic, England, Finland, France, Germany, Israel, Italy, the Netherlands), for example, indicate that close to 70% of nursing home residents have some form of cognitive impairment (Onder et al., 2012; Björk et al., 2016). Yet just 10 of 21 OECD countries reported that they can use administrative data to identify people with dementia in long-term care facilities. Without the ability to identify people with dementia, it will be difficult for countries to measure outcomes or quality of care and to determine whether policies put in place to improve care are working.

4.1.1. Institutional care must adapt further to meet the needs of people with dementia

New models of institutional care are emerging that are specialised to meet the needs of people with dementia

Small-scale living communities offer an alternative to traditional nursing-home facilities and have been adopted across the OECD. These arrangements usually comprise of living environments where people with dementia share a home with other residents and staff. Such arrangements are intended to facilitate communal living and social engagement more than traditional nursing home arrangements, with a view to improving residents' quality of life and providing them with more independence than in traditional facilities. This person-centred approach expands the focus beyond basic clinical care to facilitating the social and emotional needs of people living with dementia.

Across the OECD, about 4% of people 65 and over – and more than one in ten people over 80 – live in care facilities (see Figure 4.1). While most surveyed OECD countries reported having at least some small-scale living facilities available in their country, no countries have transitioned the majority of their residential care services to this model. Most people, including those with dementia, continue to reside in more traditional facilities. Spaces in innovative facilities, including small-scale living communities, multi-generational homes, and dementia villages are limited. Moreover dementia-specialised long-term care facilities providing the latest models of care are often private. The high costs of private nursing home care frequently creates a significant barrier to access, particularly when no- or low-cost facilities are also available.

Figure 4.1. Long-term care recipients in institutions, 65 and over

% of population aged 65 and over, 2015 (or nearest year)

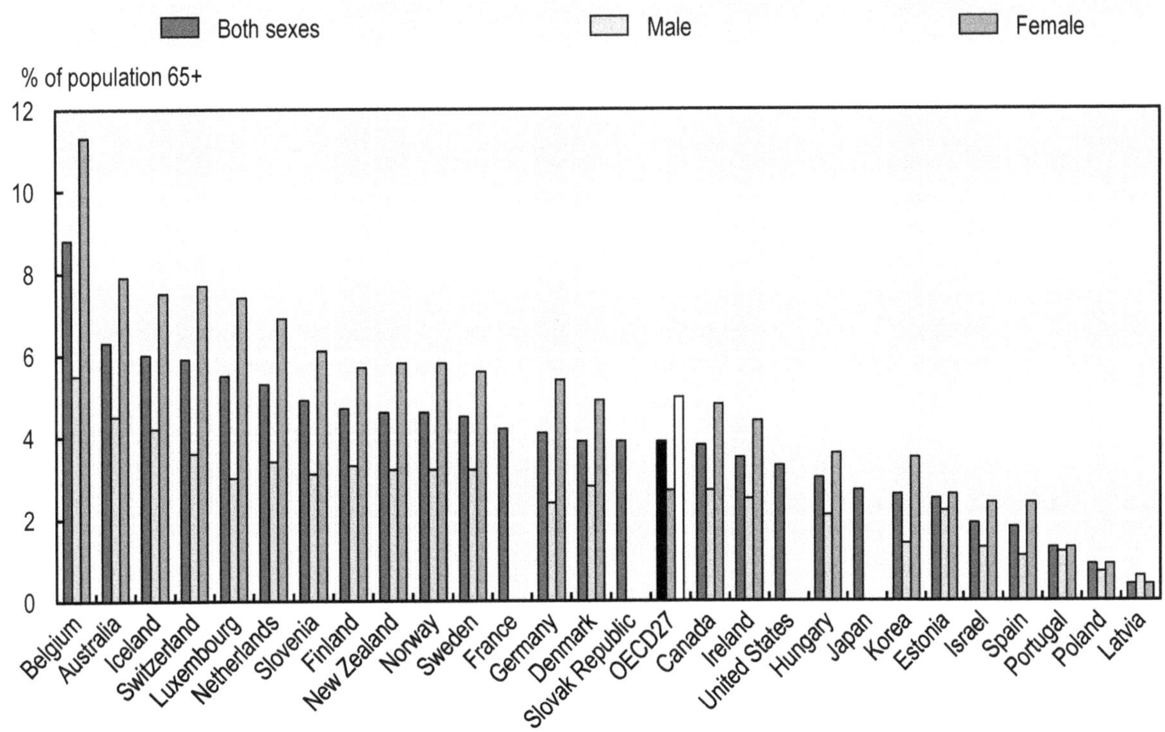

Source: *OECD Health Statistics 2017*, http://dx.doi.org/10.1787/health-data-en.

StatLink http://dx.doi.org/10.1787/888933735291

Figure 4.2. Long-term care recipients in institutions, 80 and over

% of population aged 80 and over, 2015 (or nearest year)

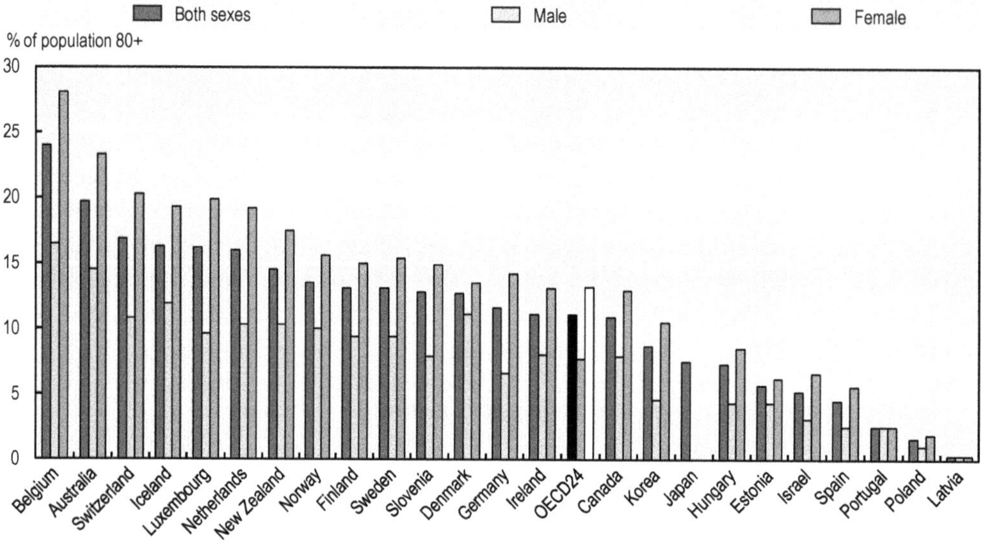

Source: *OECD Health Statistics 2017*, http://dx.doi.org/10.1787/health-data-en.

StatLink http://dx.doi.org/10.1787/888933735310

Countries should consider developing or adapting existing guidelines on dementia-friendly design to be used for new construction and renovations. The physical design of buildings can strongly impact the quality of life of people living with dementia. In more 'traditional' residential facilities, long hallways, nursing stations, and other aspects of traditional nursing home design can contribute to increased anxiety and agitation, while locked doors and other measures taken to prevent wandering can restrict autonomy and create distress. As attention to dementia has grown, a number of countries have developed design principles to incorporate into institutional care and other settings frequented by people living with dementia. Some OECD countries, including the Denmark, Ireland, Norway, and the United Kingdom (England), have developed design guidelines and advice specifically related to dementia.

Box 4.1. Improving care for people with dementia in care facilities

In 2013 and 2014, the Department of Health in England supported 42 NHS and 74 Social Care pilot projects with GBP 50 million with the goal of developing models that improve care for people with dementia. Funding was provided to range of facilities, including care facilities, hospitals, day and respite centres, general practice offices, and dementia care facilities. 73% of NHS and local authority pilot projects took place in care homes. Based on the results of the pilot studies, Loughborough University, with support from the Department of Health, developed a set of best practice guidelines on designing dementia-friendly environments. This guidance was published in 2015 as a Department of Health building note for health and social care environments.

In some cases, financing is available for or even tied to compliance with dementia-friendly design. Norway, for example, requires that residential and nursing homes built with funding from the National Bank of Housing conform to dementia-friendly design principles, while grants and subsidies are available for renovating existing homes.

More research is needed to build the evidence base on alternative models of long-term care

While the development of small-scale living facilities shows promise, more evidence on the effect of these new living arrangements on outcomes is needed. The limited research that has been conducted so far has demonstrated inconclusive though promising results in improving residents' quality of life. Studies of the 'Green House' model of small-scale group living for people with dementia in the United States have indicated that quality of life among residents of Green House communities was higher than that of residents in more traditional nursing homes, and quality of care was as good as or better than in traditional nursing homes (Kane et al., 2007). Small-scale group living facilities have been found to use far fewer restraints and psychotropic medications, a further suggestion that quality of care may be higher (Verbeek et al., 2014). Family members have also reported higher satisfaction and lower burden in small-scale group homes than traditional facilities (Lum et al., 2009, Verbeek et al., 2010). However, other evaluations have suggested no differences in the quality of life of residents in small-scale or traditional nursing facilities (Verbeek et al., 2010, Auer et al., 2017). Though the current evidence is mixed, the evidence related to higher quality of life and care is encouraging. Countries must continue to develop alternatives to traditional long-term care institutions that expand the notion of care beyond clinical improvement, to include promoting the autonomy of people living with dementia and improving their quality of life to the greatest extent possible.

4.1.2. More dementia-specific training for care staff could lead to better quality care

Substantial dementia training is rarely included in the minimum training requirements for care staff

Dementia-specific training is associated with improvements observed in how staff reacted to problems with long-term care residents (Teri et al., 2005; Spector et al., 2013). A study of Australian health care staff suggested that there were gaps in staff knowledge about dementia, particularly where they had not received specific training or cared for people with dementia (Smyth et al., 2013). Studies of training programmes delivered to formal care workers and staff members at nursing homes and other long-term care institutions indicate that dementia-specific training programmes can have a positive impact on both the staff's ability to handle difficult behaviour, and the prevalence of behavioural challenges in the first place (Livingston et al., 2005). The frequency of behavioural symptoms related to dementia have been associated with the level of staff training, among other factors, and interventions delivering staff trainings have been found to have significant impacts on reducing agitation and other behavioural challenges (Boustani et al., 2005; Chenoweth et al., 2009; Spector et al., 2013Even where professional care staff are fairly knowledgeable about dementia, there is some evidence to suggest that confidence in handling difficult situations can be low, and can be raised through dementia-specific training (Hughes et al., 2008). The level of training and experience of staff members may also impact their attitude toward people with dementia. Staff members with more training are more likely to have a positive outlook despite patient aggression, suggesting that education is helpful in changing attitudes and possibly behaviour toward people with dementia, particularly those with behavioural problems (Nakahira et al., 2009).

Formal care workers in most OECD countries are required to undergo a minimum level of training which does not always include specific information related to caring for people living with dementia. Though many OECD countries offer voluntary dementia-specific training programmes tailored for or including professional care staff, few countries have dementia-related requirements for training. Many people in care facilities have or will develop dementia, and may display behaviours that are challenging or risky to themselves and the people who care for them. Knowing how to manage these behaviours is critical to providing high quality and safe care for both people with dementia and their carers. Countries should consider how they can further incorporate dementia care into training programmes for health and social care staff, from low-skilled carers to directors of long-term care institutions. For countries that already have developed training programmes, courses can be evaluated for how well they teach components of person-centred dementia care, and additional modules considered where gaps are identified. In Australia, the move toward increasing privatisation of aged care services has incentivised aged care providers to differentiate themselves and distinguish themselves based on both available services and quality of care, including by enrolling their staff in dementia training programmes offered through Dementia Training Australia, a national government initiative implemented in partnership with universities and Dementia Australia (Box 4.2).

In some cases, dementia training is covered at least partially by basic training programmes, as in the case of training requirements to achieve different levels of qualification through the National Certificate in Health, Disability and Support in New Zealand. In Belgium, basic dementia training is required to work as a dementia-aware home-care worker. Home care organisations in Belgium must have at least some professional home workers who have received training that prepares them to provide basic home care assistance to people living with dementia. About 21 hours of in-person training is required for the position, which otherwise has a relatively low educational requirement. Since the programme was launched two years ago, more than 1 200 people have undergone training to become dementia-aware home-care workers. In Germany, a new professional care position – that of an additional care helper was established in 2009 to provide additional support in nursing homes. The position was developed out of an understanding that greater social interaction and support is important for the well-being and quality of life of people living with dementia, including those in nursing homes and other long-term care facilities. Additional care helpers are required to undergo a short training course of approximately six weeks to qualify for the position. They are not allowed to participate in direct care needs, including washing, dressing, and nursing. To incentivise participation in this new position, additional care helpers receive a special minimum wage that is higher than the legal minimum wage of each Bundeslände. Though originally developed for people with dementia, the programme was expanded in 2016 to include all people living in care homes, with a requirement that one additional care helper be available for every twenty residents.

In the United Kingdom (England), all staff members who work in organisations interacting with people with dementia are required to undergo dementia training in line with their level. The Dementia Core Skills Education and Training Framework was developed to detail the level of knowledge about dementia expected of different staff members working with people with dementia. Learning outcomes are detailed for all levels of staff, and comprise three tiers: baseline dementia awareness training (all staff); training for staff members who interact regularly with people with dementia; and training for service leaders and other experts. In addition, all health and social care staff members are required to complete at least Tier 1 dementia awareness training. Approximately 85% of social care staff have completed a care certificate for dementia, with 55% of the workforce completing a qualification of at least Tier 2.

Box 4.2. Developing national dementia training programmes in Australia

Australia offers two nation-wide training programmes for caring for people with dementia. The first, Dementia Training Australia, has made available professional dementia care development training, opportunities for upskilling, and access to accredited dementia care training courses across the country. Accredited dementia vocational courses are available at no cost to eligible care workers, including in both institutional and community-based care. Dementia Training Australia offers training opportunities across health and social professions, including courses aimed toward general practitioners, nurses and pharmacists in addition to care workers. Online training is also available. In addition, aged care providers who are interested in improving the quality of their dementia care are able to request onsite training interventions. Following an audit of the care home environment and current dementia skills, a targeted training package aimed is developed to address weaknesses identified during the audit.

The programme is run by the Australian government together with five universities and Dementia Australia. Building on programmes previously available in different parts of the country, the national platform was launched in 2016. Dementia Training Australia offers an online resource portal for health and social professionals and aged care service providers to identify available opportunities for training and accreditation.

In addition to the training opportunities offered through Dementia Training Australia, the Dementia Behaviour Management Advisory Service (DBMAS) offers assistance to both individuals and service providers when behavioural and psychological symptoms of dementia (BPSD) affects quality of life or their ability to care. DBMAS is a comprehensive, free service that offers support through a number of approaches, including individual assessment, care planning and short-term case management, mentoring, and capacity building and training for service providers.

In Denmark, nursing homes are eligible to apply for public funding to finance dementia-specific training for their staff. DKK 145 million (about EUR 19.5 million) have been allocated to support training for dementia care aides. Dementia training is similarly state-financed in Norway, where municipalities – whose memory teams offer assessment services and pre- and post-diagnostic support to people with dementia living in the community – can apply for grants to send their staff members to dementia training. The ABC dementia training programme in Norway has been found to increase knowledge about dementia and job satisfaction. Over 19 000 basic care staff have completed the programme in Norway, and similar programmes have since been adopted in other countries, including Denmark and Sweden (Box 4.3). In the Netherlands, home and institutional care workers are required to undergo basic training. The uptake of dementia-specific training programmes is largely dependent on care providers.

Box 4.3.The Dementia ABC programme in Norway

The Dementia ABC educational programme developed in Norway represents an example of how well-designed training programmes can be effectively integrated into existing health and social services to deliver high-quality care and improve job satisfaction. Developed by the Norwegian National Advisory Unit on Ageing and Health, the Dementia ABC programme is a two-year, interdisciplinary training programme open to professional staff working with people with dementia, across disciplines and levels of seniority. It is a national programme, run by the Ageing and Health unit, and works with a network of regional centres focused on dementia care education, facilitating accessibility across the country. Participants first receive informational booklets, developed by dementia care experts, which cover components of evidence-based dementia care, including engaging with both the person with dementia and their family members. Local discussion groups are organised to meet regularly to discuss the subjects discussed in the booklets and explore how these themes relate to the work of participants. Lastly, annual workshops are organised by the regional dementia care education networks. The programme was designed around a highly person-centred model of care, and emphasises the central role of the person with dementia and their families.

To promote engagement with the Dementia ABC programme, the Norwegian federal government, through the Norwegian national dementia plan, has engaged in a cost-sharing scheme with local municipalities. Municipalities pay for the informational dementia booklets and are responsible for financing the group meetings and time staff spend attending group Dementia ABC meetings. Participants in the ABC programme are compensated by their employers for the time spent attending the group meetings in about half of cases, while others attend meetings outside of their work hours. Annual workshops, which are offered twice per year, are financed through the national dementia plan.

The programme is not targeted at a specific group of professionals, but is designed to be relevant for all who may engage with people with dementia in their work lives. A longitudinal study of the Dementia ABC programme was recently undertaken using data from 90 municipalities across Norway. Of the nearly 1 800 participants included in a longitudinal survey of the programme, 26% had a bachelor's degree, 61% were auxiliary nurses with three years of high school nurse training, and 10% had no formal health or social education – representing housekeepers, gardeners, nursing assistants, and other professions. Nearly 80% of participants came from long-term care institutions, including nursing homes and special care units, with 20% providing home-based care and 2% working in day care facilities. Notably, nearly all participants – 97% – were women.

Staff members who completed the educational programme were found to have statistically significant increases in practicing person-centred care and exhibited improvements in job satisfaction. The positive effects of the programme persisted even after the educational programme was completed. Similar programmes have since been adopted in Sweden and Denmark.

Source: Rokstad et al (2016); Kristiansen (2016).

Financial incentives and certification can help encourage participation in dementia training, particularly among more junior care staff

In most cases, even where training programmes are available, health and social care professionals working with people living with dementia may lack all but personal incentives to participate. Professional caring is largely a high-stress, low-skilled and low-paid profession. Care workers may be wary of enrolling in additional training programmes at their own expense – both in terms of time and money invested – where the professional benefit of doing so is unclear. Most countries have not developed incentives for care workers to participate in skills training for dementia.

Developing recognised accreditation programmes that provide health and social care workers and service providers with a clear professional advantage can be considered by countries interested in improving their quality of dementia care. In Sweden, the Swedish Dementia Centre has launched a dementia certification programme for entire care units. Nursing homes, day care centres, hospitals, and other facilities are eligible for certification, which is achieved through an integrated training programme that focuses both on training staff in dementia competence and building strong leadership in the institution. Since the programme was launched, 56 home care units in Sweden have been certified, as has a day care centre in Germany and nursing home in Poland.

Some academic institutions have begun offering official classes and degrees in dementia care, helping to further formalise the discipline. In Australia, the University of Tasmania recently launched a series of dementia care degree programmes. Students can receive a diploma, associate's degree, or bachelor's degree through the coursework, which is conducted entirely online and can be undertaken both part- and full-time. The programme is open to people from a variety of backgrounds, including health professionals and carers. The University of Tasmania has also developed a massive open online course (MOOC) on understanding dementia. Since 2013, more than 120 000 people have enrolled in the online course, with some enrolling in dementia care degree programmes following completion.

Universities in Sweden have similarly brought dementia care into formal education with the development of a series of degree programmes. Advanced degrees in dementia care have been developed for doctors, nurses, as well as physiotherapists and occupational therapists. Dementia care study programmes have been designed as part-time programmes, to allow health professionals to continue working while undertaking advanced study. In Sweden, universities including the Karolinska Institute and Sophiahemmet University have increased the reputation of the master's degree programmes by partnering with the Stiftelsen Silviahemmet, a dementia care foundation headed by Queen Silvia of Sweden. Graduates of the programmes receive their degree and receive the title of Silvia Doctor, Silvia Occupational Therapist, Silvia Physiotherapist, or Silvia Nurse. Since the programmes were started, more than 600 nurses have completed the master's degree.

Professional care workers are typically very low paid. Few carers receive substantially more than the federally or locally-mandated minimum wage, and many work long hours, often working overtime hours with no or limited additional pay. In the United States, for example, the wages of professional care staff have been largely stagnant over the past decade, despite growing demand (PHI, 2017).

Figure 4.3. Median hourly wage by long-term care setting (United States)

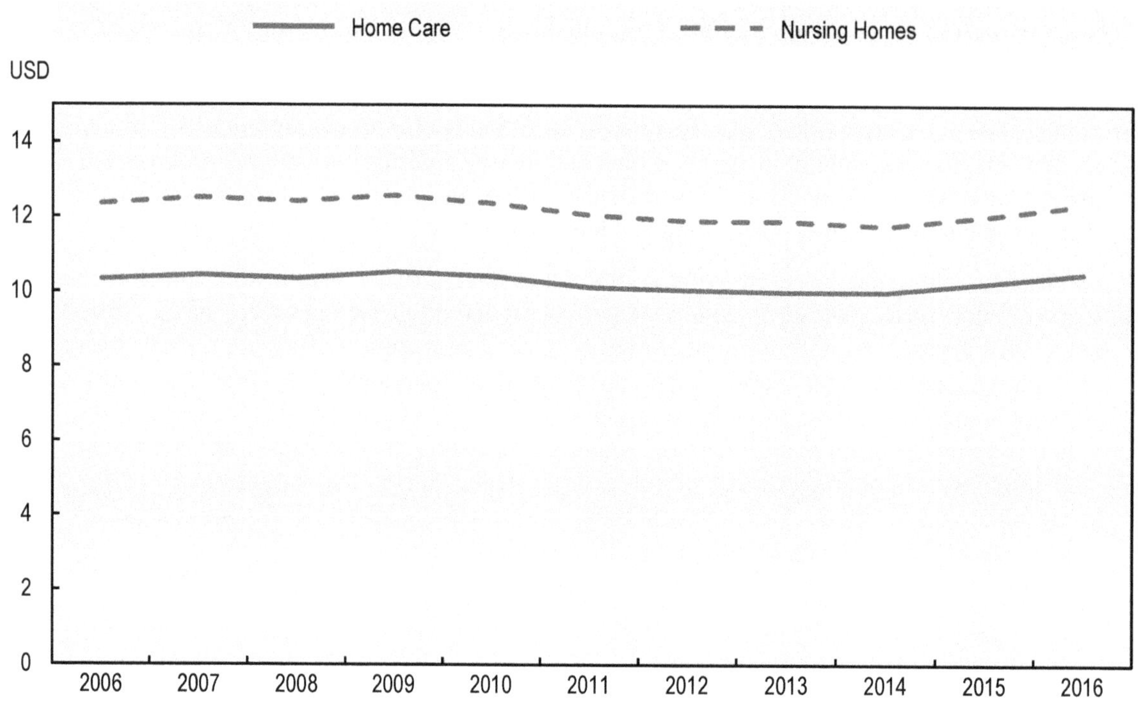

Source: PHI (2017).

StatLink http://dx.doi.org/10.1787/888933735329

Low compensation, coupled with the high stress and low social prestige of caring, often creates low job satisfaction and high turnover among carers. With the need for caring increasing with the growing elderly population, governments face opposing interests when considering how to address the issue. Raising salaries may increase the attractiveness of caring as a profession, but will also increase the costs of health and social care for governments during a time at which many are already struggling with stagnant or falling budgets.

Few countries have established salary bands for professional carers independently of applicable minimum wages. An important exception is New Zealand, where the 2017 Care and Support Workers Pay Equity Settlement Agreement has recently led to a substantial increase in the salaries of professional carers. The settlement, which resulted from a gender-discrimination claim brought by a female carer in New Zealand, has established a pay structure that sets a minimum hourly wage based on the experience of the care professional. Notably, the salary thresholds are determined by both the number of years of caring experience and the qualification levels of the carer. Carers who have achieved level 4 (senior support) of the National Certificate in Health, Disability, and Aged Support, for example, will receive a minimum salary equivalent to carers with no qualifications but 12 or more years of practical experience. These financial incentives may impact dementia care: Level 4 in the National Certificate in Health, Disability, and Aged Support receive advanced training on dementia care beyond what is taught in earlier levels of training.

Salary incentives are also in place for caregivers in Norway. Home health aides and other professional care staff will be eligible for higher salaries contingent on completion of vocational training courses focused on improving dementia care. Special minimum wage rules are also in place for additional care staff in Germany.

4.1.3. The appropriate management of behavioural and psychological symptoms of dementia (BPSD) remains a major challenge for dementia care

As the severity of dementia advances, many people living with the disease begin to experience behavioural and psychological problems, which can manifest as aggressive or agitated verbal and physical behaviour, and sometimes psychosis. Aggressive behaviours and other symptoms of BPSD have been treated by the use of physical or pharmacological restraints. This approach may prevent a person with dementia from harming themselves or others, but seriously infringes on their well-being and independence. They can also have negative health consequences: antipsychotic use can increase the risk of stroke, falls, pneumonia, and hasten cognitive deterioration (OECD, 2015a).

Despite the efforts of policymakers, the use of antipsychotics remains common and prescribing rates vary by a factor of two across OECD countries

Antipsychotic medications, which supress the behaviours by tranquilising the patient, have been frequently used to manage difficult behaviour among people living with dementia. However, many countries recommend against the practice. Antipsychotics are associated with higher mortality and a higher risk of developing strokes and other cerebrovascular events. NICE guidelines in the United Kingdom advise against administering antipsychotics to people with dementia unless they are under severe distress, or pose a risk to themselves or others. Moreover, there are ethical concerns associated with sedating people with dementia when non-pharmacological treatment options are available. Nonpharmacological interventions have furthermore been found to be effective for addressing BPSD in people with dementia (Ayalon et al., 2006). Given the widespread agreement that antipsychotic medications should not be administered to manage BPSD, rates of antipsychotic prescribing can be considered a useful indication of the quality of care people with advanced dementia are receiving. Because of difficulties in estimating the number of people living with dementia, establishing an accurate cross-national estimate of antipsychotic prescribing rates among the dementia population is challenging. Nevertheless, evidence from Swedish registry data suggests that the majority of antipsychotic prescribing for people 65 and older goes to people with dementia, suggesting that the rate of antipsychotic prescribing in older populations can be considered a useful proxy measure.

Figure 4.4. Antipsychotic prescribing rates across OECD countries

Per 1 000 people aged 65 and over

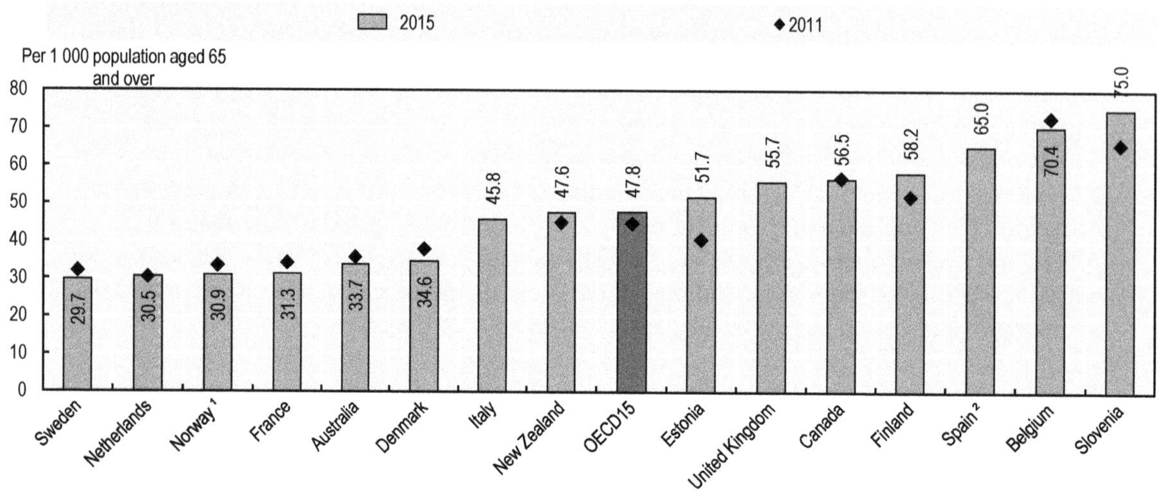

1. Data for Norway do not include people in institutional care, so underestimates the use of antipsychotics.
2. Data for Spain refer to 2014.
Source: *OECD Health Statistics 2017*, http://dx.doi.org/10.1787/health-data-en.

StatLink http://dx.doi.org/10.1787/888933735348

Across the OECD, prescribing rates for antipsychotic medications in the population aged 65 and over varies by a factor of more than two, from 30 in every 1 000 people aged 65 and over in Sweden and the Netherlands to more than 70 in Belgium and Slovenia (Figure 4.4). Encouragingly, most countries have seen prescribing rates decline over time. The majority of countries have seen stable or decreasing rates, with Denmark showing a particularly marked fall over the past eight years. While Belgium has one of the highest rates of prescription of antipsychotics, the last two years have seen a reduction from 73 per 100 people to 70. However, Slovenia shows a different pattern to other countries, with the use of antipsychotics rising steadily from 63 per 1 000 persons 65 and above in 2009 to 75 per 1 000 in 2015 – a 20% increase. This could raise concerns about the overuse of these drugs to manage difficult behaviour in older people.

Antipsychotic prescribing rates also show a marked difference between men and women. In every country surveyed, women were prescribed antipsychotics more frequently than men. In Slovenia, the prescription rate among women 65 and over was more than 50% higher than among men in the same age group (Figure 4.4). Differences in prescribing rates by sex do not appear to be driven by the age structure of women and men. In 14 of the 15 countries that reported data, women had a higher rate of antipsychotic prescribing in every five-year age group 65 and above. The only exception was the Netherlands, where women aged 80 and over had a lower prescription rate for antipsychotics than men in the same age group.

Figure 4.5. Antipsychotic prescribing rates, by sex

Per 1 000 people aged 65 and over, 2015 (or nearest year)

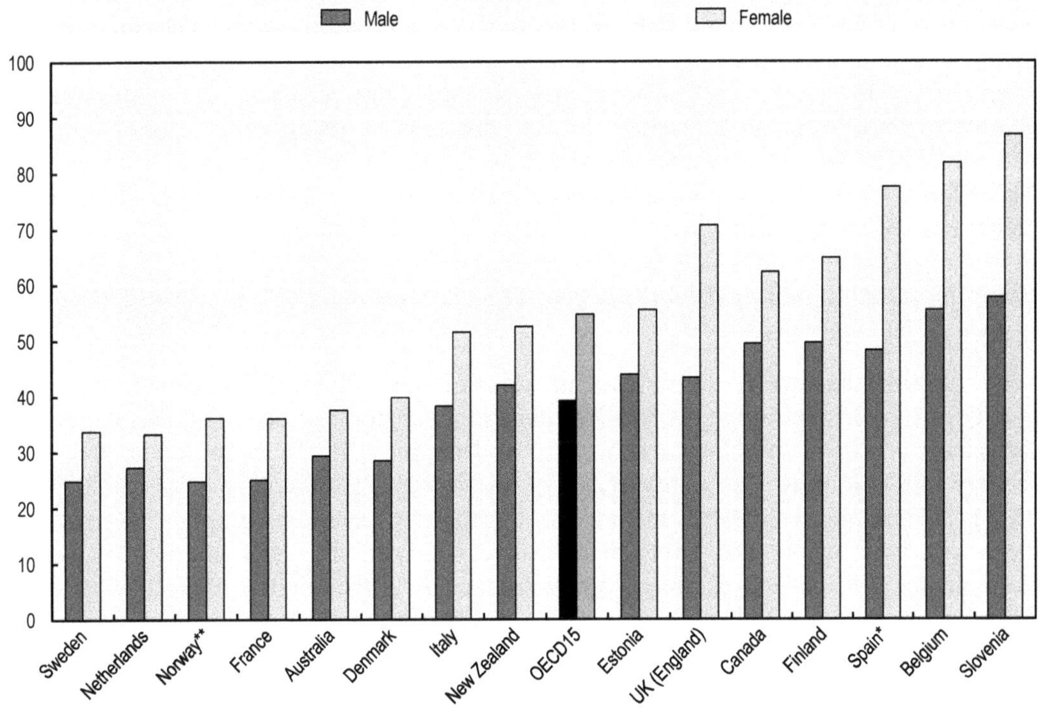

1. Data for Norway do not include people in institutional care, so underestimates the use of antipsychotics.
2. Data for Spain refer to 2014.

Source: *OECD Health Statistics 2017*, http://dx.doi.org/10.1787/health-data-en.

StatLink http://dx.doi.org/10.1787/888933735367

Beyond the work on antipsychotics, there is limited internationally-comparable data on quality indicators in long-term care. One recent effort to compare the prevalence of quality of care measures in nursing homes and hospitals has used point prevalence studies to compare the prevalence of different measures of quality in long-term care facilities, including the use of restraints. Results from the Netherlands and Austria suggest that the prevalence of physical restraints use in nursing homes remains high, at over 25% in both countries in 2012 (Halfens et al., 2013). Taken together, the recent findings on antipsychotic usage and the use of physical restraints in the Netherlands and Austria indicate that the quality of care in nursing homes remains suboptimal for many people, including those with dementia.

Some countries have developed guidelines or regulations around the use of restraints and antipsychotics

A number of OECD countries have explicitly banned or regulated the use of restraints in institutional care settings. Financial incentives may help to encourage compliance with regulations. In the United States, funding for nursing homes and other long-term care institutions from the Centers for Medicare and Medicaid Services is tied to adhering to rules related to restraints and locked wards.

Training of health and social care professional staff can also reduce the use of restraints. Staff who have been trained in alternatives to managing behavioural and psychological symptoms of dementia have been found to significantly reduce their use of restraints in institutional settings (Testad et al., 2005; Köpke et al., 2012). Less experienced staff members have also been found to have a more positive view on restraints (Hamers et al., 2008). These findings together suggest that developing clear guidelines and training programmes to teach staff alternatives to applying physical or administering pharmacological restraints can have a positive impact on the quality of life of people living with dementia. Moreover, switching away from a restraint-based approach to managing BPSD has not been found to increase suboptimal outcomes, such as increases in falls or higher rates of antipsychotic prescribing (Gulpers et al., 2011; Koczy et al., 2011).

Better monitoring of how difficult dementia symptoms are managed could help to reduce inappropriate care

Some countries have begun to monitor measures of care to inform practice and improve quality of care. In addition to the SveDem dementia registry, Sweden maintains a registry for behavioural and psychological symptoms of dementia (BPSD). Launched in 2010, the registry aims to improve the quality of care of people with BPSD in nursing homes (BPSD, 2017). All persons with BPSD included in the register have demographic information, diagnostic information, and BPSD-related care information – particularly the use of pharmacological and non-pharmacological treatments – recorded, with follow-up data recorded at multiple points. The registry facilitates continuous learning and care improvement for care professionals, including providing advice to staff on improving care based on the information entered into the registry (Sweden National Quality Registers, 2016). The registry has contributed to declines in inappropriate use of antipsychotics to manage BPSD, an important component of quality dementia care. Nearly 28 000 individuals have been included in the registry since its inception (Sweden National Quality Registers, 2016). More than half of qualifying nursing homes, care units, and BPSD teams participate in the registry (Emilsson et al., 2015).

4.2. Improving the quality of hospital care

4.2.1. Hospitals in OECD countries are not well adapted to the needs of people with dementia

Dementia is a fatal condition, with a trajectory that progresses even when care is good and all available treatments are administered. This means that even under ideal circumstances, there will be people with dementia who will need to be admitted to acute hospitals for care. Even with excellent community-based care and programmes to reduce or delay hospital admissions, people with dementia will visit hospitals, and the relevant services should be prepared to treat them when they do.

Hospitals are not always well equipped to provide people with dementia with high-quality care. Being admitted to hospital can be a distressing experience under the best of circumstances. For people with dementia, and particularly those with advanced dementia, a visit to the hospital can worsen health outcomes, and they may leave the hospital doing more poorly than when they arrived. For many hospitals, the high proportion of hospitalised patients who have dementia means that improving care for dementia patients is critical to the hospital system as a whole. In England, for example, a quarter of the hospital population is estimated to have dementia.

Outcomes for people with dementia who go into hospital are often poor

Staying in hospital can hasten cognitive and functional decline: people with dementia admitted to hospital have been found to have higher long- and short-term mortality rates than similar populations admitted to hospital who do not have dementia (Sampson et al., 2009; Morrison and Siu, 2000; Nightingale et al., 2001). These differences in outcomes between people with dementia and similar populations do not appear to be fully explained by the physical state of people with dementia. Rather, both the hospital environment and differences in the quality of care received by people with dementia appear to contribute to worse outcomes for people living with dementia. People with dementia have also been found to receive fewer palliative care treatments in hospital at the end of life than similar patients without dementia (Sampson et al., 2006).

With the negative effects of staying in hospital on people with dementia well-documented, many initiatives have focused on reducing the length of stay as much as possible. In the Netherlands, an initiative to reduce length of stay for people with dementia has adopted a "hospital at home" model for all but the most necessary treatment is in the process of being rolled out on a national level. Under this programme, people with dementia are admitted only for immediate treatment, such as surgery, with all possible follow-up conducted at home under the care of specialist nurses. Studies of hospital-at-home programmes have found that such programmes can lower the length of stay in hospital and reduce overall costs while delivering care of equal quality to acute hospital settings (Leff et al., 2005, Shepperd et al., 2009). For hospital at home to be effective, however, programmes may require intensive nursing and physician support, and strong communication and co-ordination links between community- and hospital-based care.

National audits of the hospital system can help to establish a baseline of care quality for dementia

Countries should consider undertaking national or regional reviews to help develop a baseline of the state of hospital care for people with dementia and identify key areas for improvement. In recent years, the United Kingdom, Ireland, and Switzerland have undertaken audits or investigations of hospital care quality for people with dementia, the results of which have fed into policy recommendations and changes. Results from the audits underscore how far hospitals still have to go in ensuring they deliver high-quality care for people with dementia. In Ireland, results of the 2013 hospital audit revealed that 94% of hospitals did not have a dementia care pathway in place, and that no hospitals required staff to undergo dementia awareness training (though such training was offered in about half of hospitals to doctors and nurses). 43% of patients had a mental status assessment noted in their health care records. In the United Kingdom, repeated audits of hospitals for dementia care quality have allowed them to track progress over time. They recently published the results of the third hospital dementia audit, which indicated that while progress has been made across a range of domains, further improvements can be made, including related to communication and information sharing, leadership, management of delirium, and person-centred care. National hospital audits have helped to inform policy development in both Ireland and the United Kingdom, and can serve as a model for other countries interested in improving hospital care for people with dementia.

4.2.2. Some countries are trying to improve the ability of hospital staff to effectively manage dementia

Staff training and key staff positions can help improve dementia care in hospitals

Studies of hospital staff indicate that the attitudes of health professionals, including nurses, significantly affect the care received by people living with dementia (Moyle et al., 2008; Dewing and Dijk, 2016). Many of the behavioural challenges of dementia, which can be exacerbated by the distress at being in hospital, can be difficult for hospital staff to manage effectively, and may contribute to higher levels of stress and burnout among staff members and poorer quality care, including unnecessary sedation, for people with dementia (Dewing and Dijk, 2016). Staff often report feeling under-trained in caring for dementia. This is particularly true among nurses and health care assistants, who spend more time with the patient than physicians, and may consequently impact the patient's hospital experience more directly (Gandesha et al., 2012).

Given that hospital stays can be distressing for dementia patients, and can lead to lasting deterioration in their condition, hospitals in some OECD conditions have been looking for ways to improve the care experience. A number of countries have developed innovative new staff positions and teams working in hospitals to deal specifically with patients exhibiting symptoms of dementia. In Australia, the Dementia Behaviour Management Advisory Service is available in acute hospital settings to help deal with people with dementia exhibiting behavioural and psychiatric symptoms of dementia. In Ireland, a dementia nurse specialist role has been developed in acute hospital settings to serve as a link between hospital and community-based services. A similar role has been introduced in hospitals in Slovenia. Specialist mental health liaison teams in the United Kingdom serve a similar role, and help advise hospital staff on recognising and responding to delirium and dementia.

The emergence of new specialist roles to facilitate care for people with dementia may improve the quality of care received in hospital and help ease transitions between care settings. However, countries should be careful to introduce these new positions as an addition to, rather than replacement for, improving staff training in hospitals more broadly. These positions may often serve in a responsive crisis management role, rather than contributing to a broader shift in the approach to caring for people with dementia (Holmes et al., 2010; Dewing and Dijk, 2016).

Staff training initiatives for dementia available for hospital staff members are important in improving the hospital response to dementia. In Sweden, an internet-based training module targeted specifically at hospital staff was developed by the Swedish Dementia Centre, and has made the dementia certification programme available to hospitals in addition to other care units. In England, all hospital staff are required to undergo Tier 1 dementia awareness training according to the Dementia Core Skills Education and Training Framework, while staff members who more regularly interact with patients with dementia or direct services are required to have more advanced (Tier 2 and Tier 3) training on dementia. Very few countries reported a specific focus on improving the capacity of hospital staff to care for people with dementia. In most countries, initiatives have depended much more on the initiative of individual hospitals than country- or regional training programmes. Furthermore, even where training initiatives may be open to hospital staff, practical barriers, including cost, time away from work, and lack of professional incentives can hamper participation.

Delirium is a major driver of long hospital stays and poor outcomes and could be better managed

There is some evidence to suggest that interventions targeting delirium, frailty and other geriatric conditions that are not limited to people with dementia can have positive effects on the quality of care and outcomes for people with dementia in hospitals. Delirium is a major driver of longer lengths of stay in hospital, and many people with dementia will develop the condition upon entry into hospital (Ely et al., 2001; Fick et al., 2013). The presence of delirium is a strong predictor of worse outcomes among people with dementia (Morandi et al., 2014). Some estimates indicate that between 30-60% of elderly patients have both dementia and delirium while in hospital, meaning that interventions targeting delirium will impact a high proportion of people with dementia in hospital (Saravay et al., 2004). In some countries, including Switzerland, the United Kingdom, Australia, and New Zealand, national guidelines or in-hospital protocols for delirium mitigation have been developed. The presence of standardised protocols of care for people with dementia has been found to positively impact the quality of care received acute hospitals (Moyle et al., 2008).

Countries should encourage hospitals to develop training programmes and care pathways that help to minimise the prevalence and impact of delirium on patients. A number of models have been tested and validated in multiple health care systems, most notably the Hospital Elder Life Program intervention for preventing delirium and functional decline. HELP combines staff and volunteer training with a standardised intervention protocol and continual performance tracking mechanisms to ensure quality and compliance (Inouye et al., 2000; Rubin et al., 2011). Originally piloted in the United States, HELP has since been expanded to sites in eleven countries, including Australia, the Netherlands, Italy, and Japan (Hospital Elder Life Program, 2017).

Special care units can be helpful, but may not be able to treat all people with dementia needing hospital care

Special care units and geriatric hospital wards can offer older patients with dementia more highly specialised or intensive care than they might receive in a normal ward. Recognising the special care needs of older populations, many acute care hospitals have developed geriatric and sometimes special care units to care for elderly patients. Staff members working on geriatric wards are more highly trained in geriatric issues, including dementia and delirium. Special care units, which have been developed to care for people in hospital exhibiting behavioural symptoms of dementia or delirium, are staffed by personnel who have received additional training on responding to the behavioural symptoms of dementia and delirium. In England, most hospitals have elderly care wards that are designed to support people with dementia, while a number of hospitals have also developed dementia-specialist wards. Evaluations of special care units in Australia and Germany suggest that the care received can help to reduce negative outcomes of hospitalisation, including adverse events such as falls and reductions in capacity to perform activities of daily living (ADL), though they may not reduce the length of stay in hospital (Zieschang et al., 2010; Gonski and Moon, 2012). While geriatric and special care units may help to improve outcomes for those assigned to them, the sheer number of people admitted to hospital with dementia makes it unlikely that they can serve the entire population who could benefit. Countries must therefore continue to emphasise improvements in care quality across acute hospitals more generally, and not limit their efforts to only specialised care units.

4.2.3. Inconsistent coding practices are holding back quality of dementia care and the measurement of progress in hospitals

Even where effective care interventions are put in place, the impact on outcomes for people with dementia will be limited if dementia is not recognised upon admission. Recent work by the OECD on developing comparative dementia quality indicators suggests that under-coding of dementia remains a serious challenge in nearly all OECD countries. It is unlikely that countries can reliably identify all people with dementia in hospitals. Diagnoses of dementia made in other care settings are often not effectively transferred when the patient is admitted to hospital, leaving hospitals lacking a crucial piece of medical information that can inform their approach to care. Poor coding of dementia can also make it difficult to monitor and reduce preventable hospitalisations among people living with dementia, an objective of many country strategies to improve dementia care, such as Healthy People 2020 in the United States.

Furthermore, the low dementia diagnosis rate in the population overall suggests that many people visiting hospital may not be aware that they have dementia in the first place, or may not have received a formal diagnosis that would be recorded in their medical records. In these cases, a hospital visit offers an important opportunity for patients to receive an official diagnosis of dementia and be put on the pathway towards treatment and care. Physicians, nurses and other hospital staff should therefore be trained to recognise the signs of dementia, and care pathways in hospitals should be developed that can move patients quickly from detection to diagnosis.

There is a dramatic variation in the coding of dementia between countries which cannot be explained by differences in prevalence

The challenge of under-coding dementia is made clear by the gap in dementia diagnoses recorded in hospital admissions between the admissions-based and patient-based data reported as part of the 2017 data pilot undertaken by the OECD. Coding difficulties point to a significant challenge in using administrative datasets: when datasets are standalone and not linked to the patient across health care settings, administrative data is unlikely to offer a full portrait of dementia in countries. A patient presenting in the emergency room may have a dementia diagnosis recorded in their primary care or long-term care institution record, but if this information is not available to hospital staff upon evaluation and admission, they may not be recognised or recorded as having dementia. This can affect not only the accuracy of the administrative hospital data but also the quality of care the patient may receive. Regularly linking frequently used data sets can develop a more accurate picture of dementia. In Canada, for example, the Canadian Chronic Disease Surveillance System links hospital data, physician billing, drug data and health insurance registry, covering 97% of the population. It has tracked cases of dementia through the health system since 2002-2003.

It will also be challenging to use administrative data when overall diagnosis rates are low. For example, a country with low overall diagnosis rates may report lower-than-average admissions of people with dementia to hospital. Reducing hospital admissions among people with dementia is a worthy policy goal and can serve as an important indicator of quality of care. However, a low admissions rate in the context of low overall diagnosis rates may in fact indicate the opposite. Where overall diagnosis rates are low, the number of people recorded in hospital as having dementia will also be lower. Yet in these contexts, people with dementia likely receive less and possibly worse care than in health systems where concerted efforts to improve detection of dementia have led to more people receiving the care they need.

While admissions-based data identifies only people who had dementia recorded during a specific hospital visit, patient-linked data allows researchers to tie previous hospital visits to the same patient through the use of a unique patient identifier (UPI). This can help to identify more cases of patients who have received a diagnosis of dementia in the past, but who did not necessarily have dementia recorded on their latest hospital visit. Looking at hospital admissions which included a diagnosis of dementia as a proportion of all hospital admissions, up to a third of admissions included in the patient-based version of the indicator did not have a diagnosis of dementia recorded when they entered the hospital, even though they had previously been diagnosed. In France, for example, using patient-linked data resulted in the number of admissions with a diagnosis of dementia more than doubling. This indicates that there are a significant number of cases in which a diagnosis of dementia is not effectively communicated to the hospital, and is therefore not recorded in the hospital record.

Figure 4.6. Proportion of all-cause hospital admissions with dementia captured in the hospital record, where dementia was recorded in previous three years, 2015

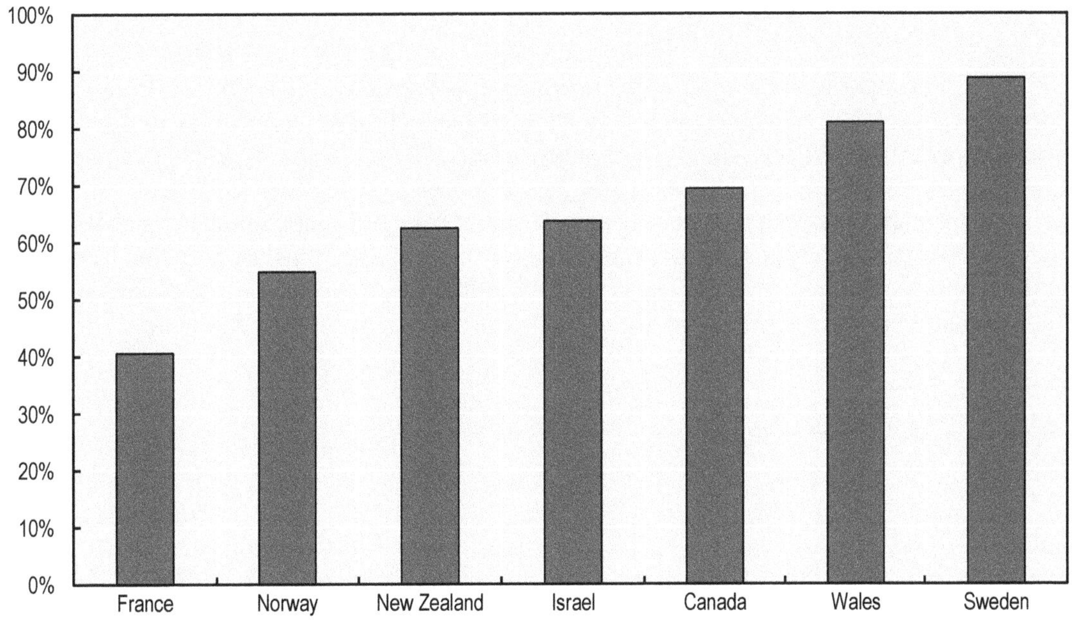

Source: OECD Dementia Care Policy Interviews 2017.

StatLink http://dx.doi.org/10.1787/888933735386

Coding guidelines for dementia could help to improve coding rates and consistency in hospitals

Further efforts should be made to improve the consistency of dementia coding in acute care, both within countries (between hospitals and regions) and ultimately internationally. Without improved coding quality in hospitals, measuring and improving quality of care is nearly impossible, as differences can be driven as much by missed cases of dementia as by real differences in the quality of care. In many countries, coding guidelines have been developed that help coders to apply international disease codes, such as the ICD-9 and ICD-10 classification list. These guidelines can differ between countries and influence how dementia is recorded on patients' medical records. In Australia, for example, dementia could previously only be coded (as either a principle or additional diagnosis) where dementia either caused the admission to hospital, or impacted care during the admission (Cummings et al., 2011). The Australian example also demonstrates how guidelines can impact dementia coding: the number of hospital admissions where dementia was recorded fell substantially following a change in coding standards in 2008. However, the decision of what constitutes an impact on care can be arbitrary, or influenced by what has previously been recorded in medical notes. More recently, a set of supplementary codes for chronic conditions, including dementia, were introduced in the 9th edition of the International Classification of Diseases, 10th revision, Australian Modification (ICD-10AM) and applies to all hospitalisation data reported since 1 July 2015. The Australian Coding Standard now states that dementia should be captured in the hospital record if present on admission, regardless of whether it was the reason for admission or required treatment. In the United Kingdom, coding guidelines were developed for general practitioners in London and the North of England after confusion over diagnostic codes was identified as a possible barrier to increasing the population in primary practice dementia registers (Russell et al., 2013). Countries should consider developing similar guidelines for applying dementia codes to hospital admissions. Doing so could help to increase the consistency in coding and ensure that possible cases of dementia do not go untreated.

Training hospital staff to recognise the symptoms of dementia may also help to improve detection and coding for dementia. It is possible that dementia is not only under-coded, but is also coded inconsistently, or only for a subset of people, such as those for whom dementia is the main reason for hospital care. Even where secondary diagnosis fields are available, physicians may not note a dementia diagnosis for an elderly patient unless accompanying symptoms, such as delirium, are present. More countries should consider adopting training interventions that improve the capacity of hospital staff working in the emergency department to recognise the symptoms of dementia, as is done in the Netherlands.

Countries are beginning to link datasets across settings, which could significantly improve the identification of dementia patients in hospitals

Of 22 OECD countries surveyed, slightly over half (13) report that they regularly link data from a minimum of four major national datasets (OECD, 2015b). However, important areas of the health system are largely excluded from data linking. Most importantly for dementia, very few countries link data systems from primary care settings (OECD, 2015b). Of 22 OECD countries, only two reported regularly linking primary care data to other pathways of health care. Including primary health data is particularly important for dementia patients given the central role primary care settings play in detecting, diagnosing, and caring for people with dementia. Where diagnosis is made by a primary care physician – as is the case for a majority of people with dementia in many countries – the exclusion of primary care from broader data linkages suggests that a patient's diagnosis may not be regularly or accurately communicated when they go to access other parts of the health system.

Figure 4.7. Number of countries reporting national data used to conduct record-linkage projects on an occasional and on a regular basis

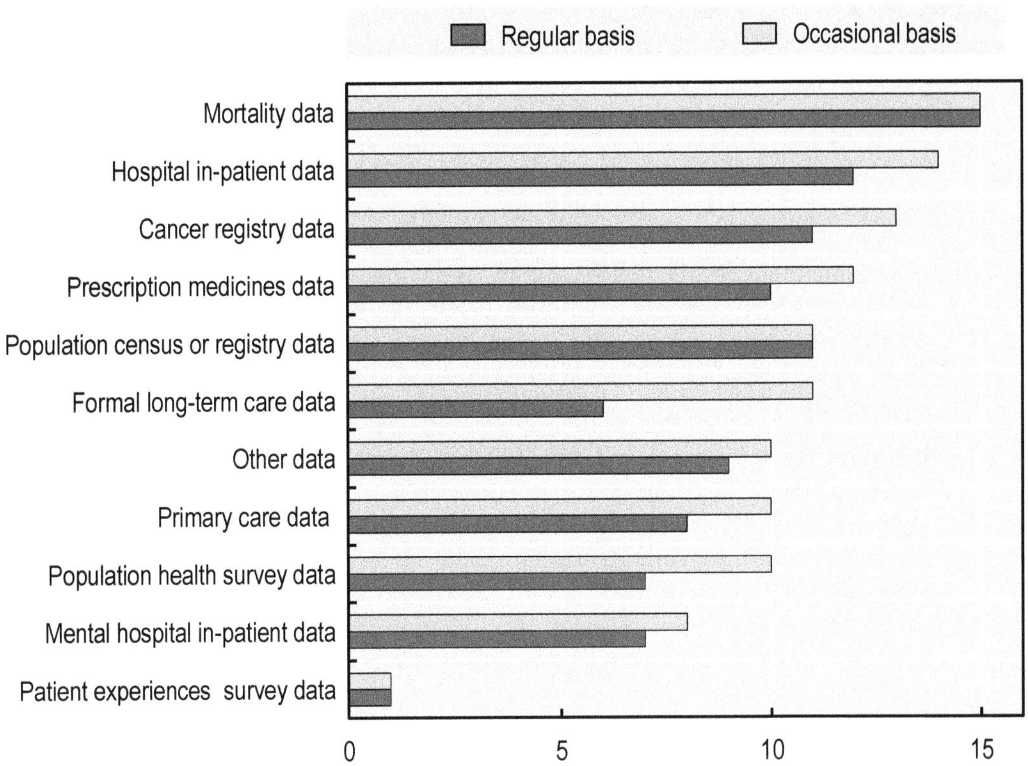

Source: OCED HCQI Questionnaire, Secondary Use of Health Data, 2011/12.

StatLink http://dx.doi.org/10.1787/888933735405

Countries must do more to improve hospital care for people with dementia

Many people with dementia will spend at least some time in an acute hospital, and it is important that hospitals are able to care for them in a way that minimizes the stress of a hospital setting. But in most countries, it is far from clear that hospitals can accurately identify all or even most people with dementia who seek care. The results of the pilot data analysis from the OECD demonstrates how in many countries, even people who had previously received a dementia diagnosis did not have this information recorded when they went to hospital. This can affect not only the accuracy of hospital data, but also the quality of care the patient receives. Coding standards that instruct health professionals on how to code diagnoses can impact how often diseases are recorded in hospital records. Because of the impact that dementia can have on even unrelated diseases, people who have been previously diagnosed with dementia should always have that information recorded in new care settings, and particularly when they visit acute hospitals. Countries should make sure that coding standards that do not impede recording dementia are in place.

4.3. Dying well: End of life and palliative care

Across OECD countries, people living with dementia continue to have insufficient access to palliative care at the advanced stages of the disease. In most countries, the palliative care model has been developed around care for cancer, a disease with a very different trajectory and end of life process than dementia. Because dementia is a terminal illness, much of the care process following a dementia diagnosis can, or should, adopt a palliative care approach, with an emphasis on person-centredness and delivering supportive rather than curative care. For the purposes of this section, however, the focus is more narrow, and examines how end-of-life palliative care is delivered to reduce pain and discomfort at the end-of-life stage of dementia (Box 4.4).

Box 4.4. What is palliative care?

According to the WHO, palliative care "is an approach that improves the quality of life of patients and their families facing the problem associated with life-threatening illness, through the prevention and relief of suffering by means of early identification and impeccable assessment and treatment of pain and other problems, physical, psychosocial and spiritual"(WHO, 2017).

Based on this and other definitions of palliative care, much of the care process for someone living with dementia can be considered to be providing palliative care, in the sense that care given to people with dementia is focused not on curing the disease, but in improving a person's quality of life and comfort to the greatest extent possible for the rest of their life. For the purpose of this chapter, palliative care is used in the context of end of life palliative care to refer to the steps taken to maximise comfort and reduce pain at the advanced and end of life stages of dementia.

4.3.1. Advance care planning is important for people with dementia, but uptake remains low

Information about what advance care planning and palliative care options should be made available to people with dementia and their families and carers in a timely manner. In the majority of countries interviewed for this report, some form of advance care planning (ACP) is available to people living with dementia. Even where advance care planning services are technically available, however, uptake appears to be low. This continues to be the case even where palliative care is covered as part of the standard basket of health services, such as in Israel. Estimates of how often advance care planning is used are unavailable in most countries, though the first national prevalence study is currently underway in Australia, while in New Zealand, all persons who receive a home care package undergo an InterRAI assessment and have their advance care planning status recorded.

Many countries reported that while advance care planning can be introduced as part of post-diagnostic care, the frequency with which physicians and care workers raise the issue with people with dementia and their families is unclear. This is true even when advance care planning is part of clinical guidelines for dementia care, as is the case in Australia and the United Kingdom (England). Advanced directives for medical care have allowed people in the United Kingdom to refuse in advance specified medical treatments under the Mental Capacity Act (2005). However, the use of advanced directives is believed to be very low, and is estimated at about 4% in England, and 2% in Wales (YouGov, 2013).

Box 4.5. What is advance care planning?

Most broadly, advance care planning refers to discussion and planning of a person's future living and care that takes place in anticipation of future physical or mental deterioration that would make communicating their wishes difficult. Some outcomes of advance care planning, including advance directives (AD) and power of attorney, are binding decisions that family members, caregivers, and health professionals are legally obligated to respect. Advance care planning may also entail non-legally binding decisions, including statements of wishes, or communication to family members and caregivers about what their future preferences would be. By helping to stimulate discussion and acceptance of the ultimate course of dementia, the advance care planning process is sometimes seen as more useful than any documents that may result (Sampson, 2010).

The decisions made during the advance care planning process are not necessarily legally binding. However, most OECD countries have developed legally-binding mechanisms that allow people with dementia to develop directives for care or appoint family members or others to serve as their financial or health care proxy (Table 4.1). In countries where legally binding advance directives are not available, physicians will have the final say on whether or not to respect the wishes conveyed by the person with dementia.

4.3.2. Palliative care for people with dementia poses specific challenges and countries should consider developing dementia-specific guidelines

Compared with cancer and other diseases, people with dementia have been found to receive notably less palliative care treatment at the end of life (Sampson et al., 2006). Patients with dementia receiving care in acute hospitals receive less palliative medication and fewer referrals to specialist palliative care than similar patients without a dementia diagnosis (Sampson et al., 2006). One study found that among patients who were admitted to hospital with a hip fracture, those with dementia received only one-third of the pain relief received by patients without dementia (Morrison and Siu, 2000).

Most notably, referrals to palliative care continue to be driven by cancer. In the United Kingdom (England, Wales and Northern Ireland), cancer caused 29% of deaths in 2012, but represented 88% of inpatient palliative care, and 75% of outpatient palliative care referrals (Dixon et al., 2015). Even as countries have begun making efforts to expand palliative care services to other conditions, cancer patients continue to be the primary beneficiaries of palliative care. Without reducing the availability of palliative care treatments for people with cancer, countries must make end-of-life palliative care more widely available to people living – and dying – with other disease.

While palliative care is available across the OECD, at least nine countries reported that it is unavailable or difficult to access for people with dementia. There is also a pressing need to make palliative care programmes more accommodating to the unique needs of people with dementia. In most countries, the development of palliative care systems has been based on the care trajectory of cancer. Providing palliative care to people with dementia can present different complications that should be taken into account. The inability of people with advanced dementia to communicate their level of pain can affect the pain relief they receive during their last months of life (Sampson, 2010). Difficulties in communicating their needs can drive people with dementia to exhibit behavioural challenges that can then result in further inappropriate care, such as the use of antipsychotics to control aggressive behaviour (OECD, 2015a). Even where specialists have been trained in palliative care, they may be less familiar with the complexities of the end of life in people with dementia.

Table 4.1. Availability of legally-binding advance care planning mechanisms

	Advance directive	Power of attorney (legal proxy)
Australia	Yes	Yes
Austria	Yes	Yes
Belgium	Yes	Yes
Czech Republic	Yes	Yes
Denmark	Yes	Yes
Estonia	Yes	Yes (financial proxy only)
Finland	Yes	Yes
France	Yes	Yes
Germany	Yes	Yes
Greece	No	Yes (financial proxy only)
Hungary	Yes	Yes
Ireland	Yes	Yes
Israel	Yes	Yes
Italy	No	Yes (financial proxy only)
Latvia	Yes	Yes
Luxembourg	Yes	Yes
Mexico	Yes (12 states + Mexico City)	
Netherlands	Yes	Yes
New Zealand	Yes	Yes
Norway	No	Yes (financial proxy only)
Poland	No	Yes
Portugal	Yes	Yes
Slovak Republic	No	Yes
Slovenia	Yes	Yes
Spain	Yes	Yes (financial proxy only)
Sweden	No	Yes (financial proxy only)
Switzerland	Yes	Yes
Turkey	Yes	Yes (health care proxy only)
United Kingdom	Yes	Yes
United States	Yes	Yes

Source: OECD Dementia Care Policy Interviews 2017; Alzheimer Europe 2017.

The development of guidelines outlining the use of palliative care among people with dementia has been demonstrated to increase the use of palliative care. The implementation of multidisciplinary guidelines on palliative care for people with dementia in the United Kingdom significantly reduced the use of antibiotics and increased the administration of pain relief during the last two weeks of life in a psychiatric hospital (Lloyd-Williams and Payne, 2002). Care staff and health workers may be unclear about the symptoms of dying in people with dementia, or uncertain about how palliative care should be applied when people are unable to communicate or clearly demonstrate they are in pain. The development of guidelines and frameworks for administering palliative care to people with dementia could help to streamline and institutionalise the use of palliative care at the end of life. No countries have developed national frameworks for administering palliative care to people with dementia, though a limited number have identified people with dementia as a target population for increasing access to palliative care.

The availability of palliative care services varies widely between countries, though in nearly all cases, the majority of palliative care places are located in tertiary hospitals. In some countries, including Denmark, Mexico and Slovenia, palliative care is not available to people with dementia who live at home. Providing palliative care at home or in a familiar environment may cause less distress for dementia sufferers and their carers and families.

In the United Kingdom, the government has committed to promoting high quality and personalised end of life care, including end of life care delivered at home and in care facilities. To improve end of life care for residents of care facilities, best practice and key lessons have been disseminated through an Enhanced Health in Care Homes framework, as well as a series of best practices published by Public Health England in 2017. Guidance published in May 2017 focuses specifically on how care staff should approach care planning for people with dementia, including examples of best practice.

In some cases, payment systems have created unnecessary barriers to accessing palliative care for people with dementia. Reimbursement practices in health systems should be reviewed to ensure that people with dementia can have end-of-life services reimbursed in a straightforward manner. In the United States, hospice care is only accessible upon receiving a prognosis of dying within six months, with only 30 days of hospice reimbursed by Medicare. People with dementia may cycle multiple times through hospice care and nursing homes as they live beyond their initial prognosis and overstay the hospice period funded by Medicare. In other countries, including Germany and the Netherlands, dementia may not always be classified as a terminal disease, creating payment challenges at the end of life when services designated for terminal patients – including palliative care and hospice – are needed (Davies et al., 2014).

4.3.3. Helping people with dementia at the end of life

The difficulties in understanding and communicating that accompany advanced stages of dementia makes meeting the needs of people with dementia at the end of life particularly difficult. Promoting advance care planning options that encourage difficult end-of-life discussions to occur before people with dementia have lost their cognitive function and ability to communicate can help them to convey their preferences before it is too late. Expanding palliative care programmes is also important to ensuring people with dementia do not experience unnecessary pain or discomfort at the end of life. Countries should ensure that existing palliative care systems adequately cover people with dementia. Where this is not the case, palliative care policies, including reimbursement policies and the location of palliative care services, should be reconsidered to ensure people with dementia at the end of life can access the services they need.

References

Auer, S. et al. (2017), "Wohngemeinschaft versus traditionelles Pflegeheim für Personen mit Demenz", pp. 1–10. https://doi.org/10.3936/1476.

Ayalon, L. et al. (2006), "Effectiveness of Nonpharmacological Interventions for the Management of Neuropsychiatric Symptoms in Patients With Dementia", *Archives of Internal Medicine*, Vol. 166, No. 20, pp. 2182–2187. https://doi.org/10.1001/archinte.166.20.2182.

Björk, S. et al. (2016), "Exploring the prevalence and variance of cognitive impairment, pain, neuropsychiatric symptoms and ADL dependency among persons living in nursing homes; a cross-sectional study", *BMC Geriatrics*, Vol. 16, No. 1. https://dx.doi.org/10.1186%2Fs12877-016-0328-9.

Boustani, M. et al. (2005), "Characteristics Associated With Behavioral Symptoms Related to Dementia in Long-Term Care Residents", *The Gerontologist*, Vol. 45, No. Special Issue 1, pp. 56–61, https://doi.org/10.1093/geront/45.suppl_1.56.

Chenoweth, L. et al. (2009), "Articles Caring for Aged Dementia Care Resident Study (CADRES) of person-centred care, dementia-care mapping, and usual care in dementia: a cluster-randomised trial", *The Lancet Neurology*, Vol. 8, No. 4, pp. 317–325. https://doi.org/10.1016/S1474-4422(09)70045-6.

Commings, E. et al. (2011), "Hospital coding of dementia: is it accurate?", *Health Information Management Journal*, Vol. 40, No. 3, pp. 5-11.

Davies, N. et al. (2014), "Quality palliative care for cancer and dementia in five European countries: some common challenges", *Aging & Mental Health*, Vol. 18, No. 4, pp. 400-410, https://doi.org/10.1080/13607863.2013.843157.

Dewing, J. and S. Dijk (2016), "What is the current state of care for older people with dementia in general hospitals? A literature review", *Dementia*, Vol. 15, No. 1, pp. 106–124. https://doi.org/10.1177/1471301213520172.

Dixon, J. et al. (2015), "Equity in the Provision of Palliative Care in the UK: Review of Evidence" (pp. 1–148). London: Personal Social Services Research Unit, London School of Economics and Political Science.

Ely, E. et al. (2001), "The impact of delirium in the intensive care unit on hospital length of stay", *Intensive Care Medicine*, Vol. 27, No. 12, pp. 1892–1900. https://doi.org/10.1007/s00134-001-1132-2.

Emilsson, L. et al. (2015), "Review of 103 Swedish Healthcare Quality Registries", *Journal of Internal Medicine*, Vol. 277, No. 1, pp. 94–136. https://doi.org/10.1111/joim.12303.

Fick, D. M. et al. (2013), "Delirium superimposed on dementia is associated with prolonged length of stay and poor outcomes in hospitalized older adults", *Journal of Hospital Medicine*, Vol. 8, No. 9, pp. 500–505. https://doi.org/10.1002/jhm.2077

Gandesha, A. et al. (2012), "Adequacy of training in dementia care for acute hospital staff", *Nursing Older People*, Vol. 24, No. 4, pp. 26-31.

Gonski, P. N. and I. Moon (2012), "Outcomes of a behavioral unit in an acute aged care service", *Archives of Gerontology and Geriatrics*, Vol. 55, No. 1, pp. 60–65. https://doi.org/10.1016/j.archger.2011.06.013.

Gulpers, M. J. M. et al. (2011), "Belt Restraint Reduction in Nursing Homes: Effects of a Multicomponent Intervention Program", *Journal of the American Geriatrics Society*, Vol. 59, No. 11, pp. 2029–2036. https://doi.org/10.1111/j.1532-5415.2011.03662.x.

Halfens, R.J.G. et al. (2013), "International prevalence measurement of care problems: results", *Journal of Advanced Nursing*, Vol. 69, No. 9, https://doi.org/10.1111/jan.12189.

Hamers, J. P. H. et al. (2009), "Attitudes of Dutch, German and Swiss nursing staff towards physical restraint use in nursing home residents, a cross-sectional study", *International Journal of Nursing Studies*, Vol. 46, No. 2, pp. 248–255. https://doi.org/10.1016/j.ijnurstu.2008.06.007

Holmes, J. et al. (2010), *Liaison Mental Health Services for Older People: A Literature review, service mapping and in-depth evaluation of service models*, National Institute for Health Research Service Delivery and Organisation programme.

Hospital Elder Life Program (2018), "Hospital elder life program (HELP) for prevention of delirium", [website], http://www.hospitalelderlifeprogram.org/.

Hughes, J. et al. (2008), "Care staff working with people with dementia: Training, knowledge and confidence", *Dementia*, Vol. 7, No. 2, pp. 227–238. https://doi.org/10.1177/1471301208091159.

Inouye, S. K. et al. (2000), "The Hospital Elder Life Program: A Model of Care to Prevent Cognitive and Functional Decline in Older Hospitalized Patients", *Journal of the American Geriatrics Society*, Vol. 48,, pp. 1697–1706.

Kane, R. A. et al. (2007), "Resident Outcomes in Small-House Nursing Homes: A Longitudinal Evaluation of the Initial Green House Program", *Journal of the American Geriatrics Society*, Vol. 55, No. 6, pp. 832–839. https://doi.org/10.1111/j.1532-5415.2007.01169.x.

Koczy, P. et al. (2011), "Effectiveness of a Multifactorial Intervention to Reduce Physical Restraints in Nursing Home Residents", *Journal of the American Geriatrics Society*, Vol. 59, No. 2, pp. 333–339. https://doi.org/10.1111/j.1532-5415.2010.03278.x.

Köpke, S. et al. (2012), "Effect of a Guideline-Based Multicomponent Intervention on Use of Physical Restraints in Nursing Homes", *The Journal of the American Medical Association*, Vol. 307, No. 20, pp. 2177–2184. https://doi.org/10.1001/jama.2012.4517.

Leff, B. et al. (2005), "Hospital at Home: Feasibility and Outcomes of a Program To Provide Hospital-Level Care at Home for Acutely Ill Older Patients", *Annals of Internal Medicine*, Vol. 143, No. 11, pp. 798–808. https://doi.org/10.7326/0003-4819-143-11-200512060-00008.

Livingston, G. et al. (2005), "Systematic Review of Psychological Approaches to the Management of Neuropsychiatric Symptoms of Dementia", *American Journal of Psychiatry*, Vol. 162, No. 11, pp. 1996–2021.

Lloyd-Williams, M. and S. Payne (2002), "Can multidisciplinary guidelines improve the palliation of symptoms in the terminal phase of dementia?", *International Journal of Palliative Nursing*, Vol. 8, No. 8, pp. 371–375.

Lum, T. Y. et al. (2009), "Effects of Green House Nursing Homes on Residents' Families", *Health Care Financing Review*, Vol. 30, No. 2, pp. 35–51.

Morandi, A. et al. (2014), "Delirium Superimposed on Dementia Strongly Predicts Worse Outcomes in Older Rehabilitation Inpatients", *Journal of the American Medical Directors Association*, Vol. 15, No. 5, pp. 349–354. https://doi.org/10.1016/j.jamda.2013.12.084.

Morrison, R.S. and A.L. Siu (2000), "A Comparison of Pain and Its Treatment in Advanced Dementia and Cognitively Intact Patients with Hip Fracture", *Journal of Pain and Symptom Management*, Vol. 19, No. 4, pp. 240–248. https://doi.org/10.1016/S0885-3924(00)00113-5.

Morrison, R.S. and A.L. Siu (2000), "Survival in end-stage dementia following acute illness", *Journal of the American Medical Association*, Vol. 284, No. 1, pp. 47-52.

Moyle, W. et al. (2008), "Best practice for the management of older people with dementia in the acute care setting: a review of the literature", *International Journal of Older People Nursing*, Vol. 3, No. 2, pp. 121–130. https://doi.org/10.1111/j.1748-3743.2008.00114.x.

Nakahira, M. et al. (2009), "Attitudes toward dementia-related aggression among staff in Japanese aged care settings", *Journal of Clinical Nursing*, Vol. 18, No. 6, pp. 807–816. https://doi.org/10.1111/j.1365-2702.2008.02479.x

Nightingale, S. et al. (2001), "Psychiatric illness and mortality after hip fracture", *The Lancet*, Vol. 357, No. 9264, pp. 1264–1265. https://doi.org/10.1016/S0140-6736(00)04421-4.

OECD (2015a), *Addressing Dementia: The OECD Response*, OECD Health Policy Studies, OECD Publishing, Paris, http://dx.doi.org/10.1787/9789264231726-en.

OECD (2015b), *Health Data Governance: Privacy, Monitoring and Research*, OECD Health Policy Studies, OECD Publishing, Paris, http://dx.doi.org/10.1787/9789264244566-en.

Onder, G. et al. (2012), " Assessment of nursing home residents in Europe: the Services and Health for Elderly in Long TERm care (SHELTER) study", *BMC Health Services Research*, Vol. 12, No. 5. https://doi.org/10.1186/1472-6963-12-5.

PHI. (2017). "Workforce Data Centre", https://phinational.org/policy-research/workforce-data-center/.

Rubin, F. H. et al. (2011), "Sustainability and Scalability of the Hospital Elder Life Program at a Community Hospital", *Journal of the American Geriatrics Society*, Vol. 59, No. 2, pp. 359–365. https://doi.org/10.1111/j.1532-5415.2010.03243.x.

Russell, P. et al. (2013), "Improving the identification of people with dementia in primary care: evaluation of the impact of primary care dementia coding guidance on identified prevalence", *BMJ Open*, Vofl. 3, No. 12. http://dx.doi.org/10.1136/bmjopen-2013-004023.

Sampson, E. L. et al. (2006), "Differences in care received by patients with and without dementia who died during acute hospital admission: a retrospective case note study", *Age and Ageing*, Vol. 35, No. 2, pp. 187–189. https://doi.org/10.1093/ageing/afj025.

Sampson, E. L. et al. (2009), "Dementia in the acute hospital: prospective cohort study of prevalence and mortality", *The British Journal of Psychiatry*, Vol. 195, No. 1, pp. 61–66. https://doi.org/10.1192/bjp.bp.108.055335.

Sampson, E. L. (2010), "Palliative care for people with dementia", *British Medical Bulletin*, Vol. 96, No. 1, pp. 159–174. https://doi.org/10.1093/bmb/ldq024.

Saravay, S. M. et al. (2004), "How Do Delirium and Dementia Increase Length of Stay of Elderly General Medical Inpatients?", *Psychosomatics*, Vol. 45, No. 3, pp. 235–242. https://doi.org/10.1176/appi.psy.45.3.235.

Shepperd, S. et al. (2009), "Avoiding hospital admission through provision of hospital care at home: a systematic review and meta-analysis of individual patient data", *Canadian Medical Association Journal*, Vol. 180, No. 2, pp. 175–182. https://doi.org/10.1503/cmaj.081491.

Smyth, W. et al. (2013), "A survey-based study of knowledge of Alzheimer's disease among health care staff", *BMC Geriatrics*, Vol. 13, No. 2. https://doi.org/10.1186/1471-2318-13-2.

Spector, A., Orrell, M. and J. Goyder (2013), "A systematic review of staff training interventions to reduce the behavioural and psychological symptoms of dementia", *Ageing Research Reviews*, Vol. 12, No. 1, pp. 354–364. https://doi.org/10.1016/j.arr.2012.06.005.

Sweden National Quality Registers, (2016), *National Quality Registry for Behavioural and Psychological Symptoms of Dementia (BPSD)*, Nationella Kvalitetsregister.

Teri, L. et al. (2005), "STAR: A Dementia-Specific Training Program for Staff in Assisted Living Residences", *The Gerontologist*, Vol. 45, No. 5, pp. 686–693. https://doi.org/10.1093/geront/45.5.686.

Testad, I., Aasland, A. M. and D. Aarsland (2005), "The effect of staff training on the use of restraint in dementia: a single-blind randomised controlled trial", *International Journal of Geriatric Psychiatry*, Vol. 20, No. 6, pp. 587–590. https://doi.org/10.1002/gps.1329.

Verbeek, H. et al. (2010), "Dementia Care Redesigned: Effects of Small-Scale Living Facilities on Residents, Their Family Caregivers, and Staff", *Journal of the American Medical Directors Association*, Vol. 11, No. 9, pp. 662–670. https://doi.org/10.1016/j.jamda.2010.08.001.

Verbeek, H. et al. (2014), "Effects of small-scale, home-like facilities in dementia care on residents' behavior, and use of physical restraints and psychotropic drugs: a quasi-experimental study", *International Psychogeriatrics*, Vol. 26, No. 04, pp. 657–668. https://doi.org/10.1017/S1041610213002512

World Health Organization. (2018), *WHO Definition of Palliative Care* [website], retrieved from http://www.who.int/cancer/palliative/definition/en/.

Zieschang, T. et al. (2010), "Improving care for patients with dementia hospitalized for acute somatic illness in a specialized care unit: a feasibility study", *International Psychogeriatrics*, Vol. 22, No. 1, pp. 139–146. https://doi.org/10.1017/S1041610209990494.

ORGANISATION FOR ECONOMIC CO-OPERATION AND DEVELOPMENT

The OECD is a unique forum where governments work together to address the economic, social and environmental challenges of globalisation. The OECD is also at the forefront of efforts to understand and to help governments respond to new developments and concerns, such as corporate governance, the information economy and the challenges of an ageing population. The Organisation provides a setting where governments can compare policy experiences, seek answers to common problems, identify good practice and work to co-ordinate domestic and international policies.

The OECD member countries are: Australia, Austria, Belgium, Canada, Chile, the Czech Republic, Denmark, Estonia, Finland, France, Germany, Greece, Hungary, Iceland, Ireland, Israel, Italy, Japan, Korea, Latvia, Luxembourg, Mexico, the Netherlands, New Zealand, Norway, Poland, Portugal, the Slovak Republic, Slovenia, Spain, Sweden, Switzerland, Turkey, the United Kingdom and the United States. The European Union takes part in the work of the OECD.

OECD Publishing disseminates widely the results of the Organisation's statistics gathering and research on economic, social and environmental issues, as well as the conventions, guidelines and standards agreed by its members.

OECD PUBLISHING, 2, rue André-Pascal, 75775 PARIS CEDEX 16
(81 2018 10 1 P) ISBN 978-92-64-08509-1 – 2018

www.ingramcontent.com/pod-product-compliance
Ingram Content Group UK Ltd.
Pitfield, Milton Keynes, MK11 3LW, UK
UKHW051503290926
15471UKWH00008B/1388

9 789264 085091